2. Chicken Alfredo

Ingredient:

• 8 oz fettuccine pasta
• 2 boneless, skinless chicken breasts
• 2 tbsp olive oil
• 1/2 tsp salt
• 1/4 tsp black pepper
• 2 cups heavy cream
• 1 cup grated Parmesan cheese
• 2 cloves garlic, minced
• 2 tbsp unsalted butter
• 2 tbsp chopped fresh parsley (optional)

Instructions:

1. Bring a large pot of salted water to a boil. Add the fettuccine and cook according to package instructions until al dente. Drain and set aside.

2. Season the chicken breasts with salt and pepper. Heat the olive oil in a large skillet over medium•high heat. Add the chicken and cook for 5•7 minutes per side, until cooked through. Remove from heat and slice or shred the chicken.

3. In the same skillet, add the heavy cream, Parmesan, and garlic. Bring to a simmer and cook for 2•3 minutes, stirring frequently, until the sauce thickens slightly.

4. Reduce heat to low and stir in the butter until melted and fully incorporated.

5. Add the cooked fettuccine and shredded chicken to the sauce and toss to coat everything evenly.

6. Serve immediately, garnished with chopped fresh parsley if desired.

3. Tacos

Ingredient:

- 1 lb ground beef or ground turkey
- 1 packet taco seasoning
- 1/2 cup water
- 8•10 taco shells or soft tortillas
- Shredded lettuce
- Diced tomatoes
- Shredded cheddar cheese
- Sour cream (optional)
- Salsa (optional)

Instructions:

1. In a large skillet over medium•high heat, cook the ground beef or turkey until browned and crumbled, 5•7 minutes. Drain any excess fat.

2. Stir in the taco seasoning and water. Bring to a simmer and cook for 2•3 minutes, until the sauce has thickened.

3. Warm the taco shells or tortillas according to package instructions.

4. To assemble the tacos, layer each shell or tortilla with some of the seasoned ground meat, shredded lettuce, diced tomatoes, and shredded cheese.

5. Top with a dollop of sour cream and/or salsa, if desired.

6. Serve immediately and enjoy!

You can customize the toppings to your liking, such as adding diced onions, sliced olives, guacamole, or hot sauce. The key is the flavorful taco meat seasoned with the taco seasoning packet.

Welcome to ***"The Essential Cookbook for Men: 110+ Easy-to-Follow Recipes for Delicious Meals Any Guy Can Make"***! This cookbook is designed to equip you with the skills and recipes you need to confidently navigate the kitchen and create flavorful meals that will impress family and friends.

Embrace Your Inner Chef

Cooking isn't just about nourishment; it's a creative and rewarding experience that allows you to explore flavors, techniques, and culinary traditions. Whether you're a complete novice or a seasoned home cook looking to expand your repertoire, this book has something for everyone.

Why This Cookbook?

We understand that life can be busy, and sometimes the thought of cooking a meal from scratch can seem daunting. That's why we've curated a collection of over 110 easy-to-follow recipes that are tailored to the tastes and preferences of men. From hearty dinners to crowd-pleasing appetizers and indulgent desserts, each recipe is designed to be straightforward and achievable, even for those with limited kitchen experience.

What You'll Discover Inside

In these pages, you'll find:

- ***Simple Techniques:*** Learn essential cooking skills and techniques that will empower you in the kitchen.

- ***Flavorful Dishes:*** Explore a variety of dishes that range from classic comfort foods to contemporary culinary delights.

- ***Efficient Meal Preparation:*** Recipes that are efficient to prepare, ensuring you spend less time cooking and more time enjoying meals with loved ones.

- ***Healthy Choices:*** Discover nutritious options that prioritize fresh ingredients and balanced eating.

Embark on a journey of culinary discovery with **"The Essential Cookbook for Men"**. Whether you're looking to expand your cooking skills, impress your friends, or simply enjoy delicious homemade meals, this book is your go-to resource. Get ready to roll up your sleeves, sharpen your knives, and dive into the world of flavors waiting to be explored. Happy cooking!

1. Spaghetti and meatballs

Ingredient:

- 1 lb ground beef
- 1 cup breadcrumbs
- 1/2 cup grated Parmesan cheese
- 2 eggs, beaten
- 2 cloves garlic, minced
- 1 tsp dried oregano
- 1/2 tsp salt
- 1/4 tsp black pepper
- 1 jar (24•28 oz) marinara sauce
- 12 oz spaghetti pasta

Instructions:

1. In a large bowl, combine the ground beef, breadcrumbs, Parmesan, eggs, garlic, oregano, salt, and pepper. Mix well until fully incorporated.

2. Roll the mixture into 1•inch meatballs and place them on a baking sheet or plate.

3. In a large skillet or Dutch oven, heat the marinara sauce over medium heat.

4. Carefully add the meatballs to the sauce and gently stir to coat. Simmer for 20•25 minutes, turning the meatballs occasionally, until cooked through.

5. Meanwhile, bring a large pot of salted water to a boil. Add the spaghetti and cook according to package instructions until al dente.

6. Drain the spaghetti and serve immediately, topped with the spaghetti and meatballs in sauce.

Enjoy your classic spaghetti and meatballs!

4. Pizza

Ingredient:

Dough:
• 1 packet (2 1/4 tsp) active dry yeast
• 1 cup warm water (110°F•115°F)
• 2 1/2 cups all•purpose flour
• 1 tsp salt
• 1 tbsp olive oil

Toppings:
• 1 cup marinara or pizza sauce
• 2 cups shredded mozzarella cheese
• Desired toppings (pepperoni, mushrooms, onions, bell peppers, etc.)

Instructions:

1. Make the dough: In a large bowl, combine the warm water and yeast. Let sit for 5 minutes until foamy.

2. Add the flour, salt, and olive oil. Stir until a shaggy dough forms.

3. Turn the dough out onto a lightly floured surface and knead for 5•7 minutes until smooth and elastic.

4. Place the dough in a lightly greased bowl, cover, and let rise for 1 hour or until doubled in size.

5. Preheat oven to 450°F. Grease a pizza pan or baking sheet.

6. Punch down the dough to release air bubbles. Use your hands or a rolling pin to stretch and shape the dough into a 12•inch circle on the prepared pan.

7. Spread the sauce evenly over the dough, leaving a 1/2 inch border. Top with the shredded mozzarella and desired toppings.

8. Bake for 12•15 minutes, until the crust is golden brown and the cheese is melted and bubbly.

9. Let cool for 5 minutes, then slice and serve!

You can customize the toppings to your liking. Enjoy your homemade pizza!

5. Burgers

Ingredient:

- 1 lb ground beef
- 1 tsp salt
- 1/2 tsp black pepper
- 4 hamburger buns, split
- Desired toppings (lettuce, tomato, onion, cheese, pickles, etc.)

Instructions:

1. In a large bowl, gently mix together the ground beef, salt, and pepper until just combined. Be careful not to overmix.

2. Divide the beef mixture into 4 equal portions and shape them into patties, each about 4•5 inches wide and 1/2 inch thick. Make a slight indentation in the center of each patty with your thumb.

3. Preheat a grill or grill pan over medium•high heat.

4. Grill the patties for 3•4 minutes per side, or until they reach your desired doneness. For medium•rare, the internal temperature should reach 130•135°F. For medium, aim for 140•145°F.

5. During the last minute of cooking, toast the hamburger buns on the grill or in a toaster.

6. Place the grilled patties on the toasted buns and top with your desired toppings.

Tips:
- Use freshly ground beef for the best texture and flavor.
- Handle the meat gently to prevent the burgers from becoming tough.
- Avoid pressing down on the patties while cooking, as this can squeeze out the juices.
- Let the burgers rest for a few minutes before serving to allow the juices to redistribute.
- Customize the toppings to your liking • classics include cheese, lettuce, tomato, onion, pickles, and condiments like ketchup, mustard, and mayonnaise.

6. Stir·fry

Ingredient:

• 1 lb boneless, skinless chicken breasts, cut into 1·inch pieces
• 2 tbsp vegetable oil
• 1 cup broccoli florets
• 1 red bell pepper, sliced
• 1 cup sliced mushrooms
• 1 cup snow peas or snap peas
• 3 cloves garlic, minced
• 1 tbsp grated fresh ginger
• 2 tbsp soy sauce
• 1 tbsp rice vinegar
• 1 tsp sesame oil
• Salt and pepper to taste
• Cooked rice, for serving

Instructions:

1. Heat the vegetable oil in a large skillet or wok over high heat.

2. Add the chicken and stir·fry for 3·4 minutes, until lightly browned. Remove the chicken from the pan and set aside.

3. Add the broccoli, bell pepper, mushrooms, and snow peas to the hot pan. Stir·fry for 3·4 minutes, until the vegetables are crisp·tender.

4. Add the garlic and ginger to the pan and stir·fry for 1 minute, until fragrant.

5. Return the chicken to the pan and add the soy sauce, rice vinegar, and sesame oil. Toss everything together and cook for 2·3 minutes, until the chicken is cooked through and the sauce has thickened slightly.

6. Season with salt and pepper to taste. Serve the stir·fry immediately over cooked rice.

Tips:
• Use a variety of fresh, crisp vegetables for the best texture.
• Adjust the cooking time for the vegetables based on their firmness • harder veggies like broccoli may need a bit longer.
• Feel free to substitute the protein with beef, shrimp, or tofu.
• Add a splash of water or broth if the stir·fry seems too dry.

7. Macaroni and cheese

Ingredient:

- 8 oz elbow macaroni
- 3 tbsp unsalted butter
- 3 tbsp all•purpose flour
- 2 cups milk
- 1 tsp salt
- 1/4 tsp black pepper
- 2 cups shredded cheddar cheese
- 1/2 cup grated Parmesan cheese

Instructions:

1. Bring a large pot of salted water to a boil. Add the macaroni and cook according to package instructions until al dente. Drain and set aside.

2. In a medium saucepan, melt the butter over medium heat. Whisk in the flour and cook for 1 minute, stirring constantly.

3. Gradually whisk in the milk. Bring the mixture to a simmer and cook, stirring frequently, until thickened, about 5 minutes.

4. Remove the sauce from heat and stir in the salt, pepper, cheddar cheese, and Parmesan cheese until the cheese is melted and the sauce is smooth.

5. Add the cooked macaroni to the cheese sauce and stir to combine.

6. Transfer the macaroni and cheese to a baking dish. If desired, top with additional shredded cheese.

7. Bake at 375°F for 15•20 minutes, until the top is golden brown and bubbly.

8. Let the macaroni and cheese cool for 5 minutes before serving.

Tips:
- Use a blend of cheeses for more flavor, such as cheddar, Gruyère, and Parmesan.
- Add cooked bacon, diced ham, or sautéed vegetables for extra flavor.
- Top with breadcrumbs or crushed crackers for a crispy topping.
- Reheat leftovers in the oven or microwave.

8. Chicken nuggets

Ingredient:

• 1 lb boneless, skinless chicken breasts, cut into 1•inch pieces
• 1 cup all•purpose flour
• 2 eggs, beaten
• 1 cup panko breadcrumbs
• 1 tsp salt
• 1/2 tsp black pepper
• 1/2 tsp garlic powder
• Vegetable oil for frying

Instructions:

1. Set up a breading station with three shallow dishes: one with the flour, one with the beaten eggs, and one with the panko breadcrumbs mixed with the salt, pepper, and garlic powder.

2. Dredge the chicken pieces in the flour, dip them in the egg, and then coat them in the seasoned breadcrumbs, pressing gently to help the crumbs adhere.

3. In a large skillet or Dutch oven, heat about 1•2 inches of vegetable oil over medium•high heat to 350°F.

4. Working in batches, carefully add the breaded chicken nuggets to the hot oil and fry for 2•3 minutes per side, until golden brown and cooked through.

5. Transfer the fried chicken nuggets to a paper towel•lined plate to drain any excess oil.

6. Serve the homemade chicken nuggets warm, with your favorite dipping sauces like honey mustard, barbecue, or ranch.

Tips:
• Use chicken tenders or boneless, skinless thighs for extra juicy nuggets.
• For a healthier option, bake the breaded chicken at 400°F for 15•20 minutes instead of frying.
• Experiment with different seasoning blends in the breadcrumbs, such as Parmesan, herbs, or spices.
• Let the oil return to temperature between batches for the best frying results.

9. Grilled cheese sandwich

Ingredient:

• 2 slices of bread (white, sourdough, or your favorite)
• 2•3 slices of cheese (cheddar, American, Swiss, etc.)
• 2 tbsp butter, softened

Instructions:

1. Preheat a skillet or griddle over medium heat.

2. Spread the softened butter evenly on one side of each slice of bread.

3. Place one slice of bread, butter•side down, in the preheated skillet. Top with the slices of cheese.

4. Place the other slice of bread, butter•side up, on top of the cheese.

5. Cook the sandwich for 2•3 minutes, or until the bottom slice is golden brown.

6. Carefully flip the sandwich and cook for another 2•3 minutes, or until the cheese is melted and the second slice is golden brown.

7. Remove the grilled cheese sandwich from the skillet and let it cool for 1•2 minutes before serving.

Tips:
• Use a variety of cheeses for different flavors and textures.
• Add other ingredients like tomato, bacon, or ham for a more complex grilled cheese.
• Spread the butter all the way to the edges of the bread for a crispy, golden crust.
• Use a heavy skillet or griddle to get a nice, even cook on the bread.

10. Quesadillas

Ingredient:

• 8 flour tortillas (8•inch size)
• 2 cups shredded Monterey Jack or cheddar cheese
• 1 lb boneless, skinless chicken breasts, cooked and shredded (or use cooked ground beef/turkey)
• 1 bell pepper, sliced
• 1 onion, sliced
• 2 tbsp butter or oil
• Salsa, guacamole, sour cream for serving (optional)

Instructions:

1. Preheat a large skillet or griddle over medium heat.

2. Place one tortilla in the skillet. On one half of the tortilla, layer some of the shredded cheese, chicken (or other protein), bell pepper, and onion.

3. Fold the other half of the tortilla over the filled half to create a half•moon shape.

4. Cook the quesadilla for 2•3 minutes per side, until the tortilla is lightly browned and the cheese is melted.

5. Carefully transfer the cooked quesadilla to a cutting board. Cut it in half and repeat the process with the remaining ingredients to make 4 total quesadillas.

6. Serve the quesadillas warm, with salsa, guacamole, and sour cream on the side for dipping, if desired.

Tips:
• Use a variety of fillings like black beans, corn, jalapeños, or different cheeses.
• Brush the outside of the tortillas with a little butter or oil for extra crispiness.
• Cook the quesadillas in batches to ensure even browning.
• Keep the filled quesadillas warm in a 200°F oven while you cook the remaining ones.

11. Fried rice

Ingredient:

- 3 cups cooked and chilled white rice
- 2 tbsp vegetable oil
- 2 eggs, beaten
- 1 cup frozen peas and carrots, thawed
- 3 green onions, sliced
- 2 cloves garlic, minced
- 2 tbsp soy sauce
- 1 tsp sesame oil
- Salt and pepper to taste

Instructions:

1. Heat the vegetable oil in a large skillet or wok over medium•high heat.

2. Pour the beaten eggs into the hot pan and scramble them, breaking them up into small pieces as they cook. Remove the eggs from the pan and set aside.

3. Add the peas and carrots, green onions, and garlic to the pan. Stir•fry for 2•3 minutes until fragrant.

4. Add the chilled rice to the pan and use a spatula to break up any clumps. Stir•fry for 3•4 minutes, allowing the rice to get lightly browned.

5. Return the scrambled eggs to the pan and add the soy sauce and sesame oil. Toss everything together until well combined.

6. Season with salt and pepper to taste.

7. Serve the fried rice hot, garnished with additional green onions if desired.

Tips:
- Use day•old or chilled rice for best results • freshly cooked rice can be too sticky.
- Feel free to add other vegetables like mushrooms, bell peppers, or bean sprouts.
- For protein, you can add cooked shrimp, chicken, or diced ham.
- Adjust the soy sauce and sesame oil to your taste preferences.
- Serve the fried rice as a main dish or as a side.

12. Chicken Parmesan

Ingredient:

• 4 boneless, skinless chicken breasts
• 1 cup all•purpose flour
• 2 eggs, beaten
• 1 cup breadcrumbs
• 1/2 cup grated Parmesan cheese
• 1 tsp dried oregano
• 1/2 tsp garlic powder
• 1/2 tsp salt
• 1/4 tsp black pepper
• 2 cups marinara sauce
• 8 oz shredded mozzarella cheese

Instructions:

1. Preheat oven to 400°F. Grease a baking sheet or 9x13 inch baking dish.

2. Pound the chicken breasts between two sheets of plastic wrap or wax paper to an even 1/2•inch thickness.

3. Set up a breading station with three shallow dishes: one with the flour, one with the beaten eggs, and one with the breadcrumbs mixed with the Parmesan, oregano, garlic powder, salt, and pepper.

4. Dredge the chicken breasts in the flour, dip them in the egg, and then coat them in the breadcrumb mixture, pressing gently to help the crumbs adhere.

5. Place the breaded chicken on the prepared baking sheet or in the baking dish.

6. Bake for 15•20 minutes, until the chicken is cooked through and the breading is golden brown.

7. Top each chicken breast with about 1/2 cup of the marinara sauce and sprinkle with the shredded mozzarella cheese.

8. Return the dish to the oven and bake for an additional 5•10 minutes, until the cheese is melted and bubbly.

9. Serve the Chicken Parmesan hot, garnished with fresh basil or parsley if desired. Enjoy!

13. Lasagna

Ingredient:

- 9 lasagna noodles
- 1 lb ground beef
- 1 onion, diced
- 3 cloves garlic, minced
- 1 (24 oz) jar marinara sauce
- 1 (15 oz) can tomato sauce
- 1 tsp dried oregano
- 1/2 tsp salt
- 1/4 tsp black pepper
- 15 oz ricotta cheese
- 1 egg
- 1/2 cup grated Parmesan cheese
- 2 cups shredded mozzarella cheese

Instructions:

1. Preheat oven to 375°F. Bring a large pot of salted water to a boil. Cook the lasagna noodles according to package instructions until al dente. Drain and set aside.

2. In a large skillet over medium•high heat, cook the ground beef, onion, and garlic until the beef is browned and crumbled, about 5•7 minutes. Drain any excess fat.

3. Stir in the marinara sauce, tomato sauce, oregano, salt, and pepper. Simmer for 10 minutes.

4. In a medium bowl, mix together the ricotta cheese, egg, and 1/4 cup of the Parmesan cheese.

5. Spread 1 cup of the meat sauce in the bottom of a 9x13 inch baking dish. Arrange 3 lasagna noodles over the sauce. Spread half of the ricotta mixture over the noodles, then top with 1 cup of the meat sauce and 1/2 cup of the mozzarella cheese.

6. Repeat the layers of noodles, ricotta, meat sauce, and mozzarella. Top with the remaining 3 noodles and the remaining meat sauce.

7. Sprinkle the top with the remaining 1/4 cup Parmesan cheese.

8. Cover with foil and bake for 40 minutes. Remove the foil and bake for an additional 10•15 minutes, until the cheese is melted and bubbly. Let the lasagna cool for 10•15 minutes before slicing and serving.

14. Baked ziti

Ingredient:

- 12 oz ziti or penne pasta
- 1 lb ground beef or Italian sausage
- 1 onion, diced
- 3 cloves garlic, minced
- 1 (24 oz) jar marinara sauce
- 1 (15 oz) container ricotta cheese
- 2 cups shredded mozzarella cheese
- 1/2 cup grated Parmesan cheese
- 2 eggs
- 1 tsp dried oregano
- 1/2 tsp salt
- 1/4 tsp black pepper

Instructions:

1. Preheat oven to 375°F. Grease a 9x13 inch baking dish.

2. Bring a large pot of salted water to a boil. Cook the ziti according to package instructions until al dente. Drain and set aside.

3. In a large skillet over medium•high heat, cook the ground beef or sausage, onion, and garlic until the meat is browned and crumbled, about 5•7 minutes. Drain any excess fat.

4. Stir in the marinara sauce and simmer for 5 minutes.

5. In a large bowl, mix together the ricotta cheese, 1 cup of the mozzarella, the Parmesan, eggs, oregano, salt, and pepper.

6. Add the cooked ziti and the meat sauce to the ricotta mixture and stir to combine.

7. Transfer the ziti mixture to the prepared baking dish. Top with the remaining 1 cup of mozzarella cheese.

8. Bake for 25•30 minutes, until the cheese is melted and bubbly.

9. Let the baked ziti cool for 5•10 minutes before serving.

15. Chicken tacos

Ingredient:

- 1 lb boneless, skinless chicken breasts
- 1 packet taco seasoning
- 1/2 cup water
- 8•10 taco shells or soft tortillas
- Shredded lettuce
- Diced tomatoes
- Shredded cheddar cheese
- Sour cream (optional)
- Salsa (optional)

Instructions:

1. Place the chicken breasts in a large skillet and add the taco seasoning and water. Bring to a simmer over medium heat.

2. Cover the skillet and cook the chicken for 15•20 minutes, turning occasionally, until the chicken is cooked through and shreds easily with a fork.

3. Remove the chicken from the skillet and shred it using two forks.

4. Return the shredded chicken to the skillet and stir to coat it in the seasoned cooking liquid.

5. Warm the taco shells or tortillas according to package instructions.

6. To assemble the tacos, layer each shell or tortilla with some of the shredded chicken, shredded lettuce, diced tomatoes, and shredded cheddar cheese.

7. Top with a dollop of sour cream and/or salsa, if desired.

8. Serve the chicken tacos immediately and enjoy!

Tips:
- Use boneless, skinless chicken thighs for extra juicy and flavorful chicken.
- For a creamier taco, mix the shredded chicken with a bit of sour cream or cream cheese.
- Customize the toppings to your liking, such as adding diced onions, sliced olives, or guacamole.
- Serve the chicken tacos with additional taco toppings on the side for everyone to customize their own.

16. Pulled pork sandwiches

Ingredient:

• 3•4 lb pork shoulder or butt, trimmed of excess fat
• 1 cup barbecue sauce, plus more for serving
• 8•10 hamburger buns or brioche rolls
• Coleslaw, for serving (optional)

Dry Rub:
• 2 tbsp brown sugar
• 2 tsp smoked paprika
• 1 tsp garlic powder
• 1 tsp onion powder
• 1 tsp chili powder
• 1 tsp salt
• 1/2 tsp black pepper

Instructions:

1. In a small bowl, mix together all the dry rub ingredients. Rub the mixture all over the pork shoulder.

2. Place the seasoned pork in a slow cooker and cook on low for 8•10 hours, or until the meat is very tender and easily shreds with a fork.

3. Remove the pork from the slow cooker and transfer to a cutting board. Use two forks to shred the meat, discarding any large pieces of fat.

4. Return the shredded pork to the slow cooker and stir in 1 cup of barbecue sauce. Keep the pork on the warm setting until ready to serve.

5. Toast the hamburger buns or brioche rolls.

6. Scoop the saucy pulled pork onto the bottom buns. Top with additional barbecue sauce and coleslaw, if desired.

7. Cover with the top buns and serve immediately.

Tips:
• Use a dry rub with a blend of sweet, savory, and smoky spices for maximum flavor.
• Cook the pork in the slow cooker for hands•off convenience, or in the oven at 300°F for 3•4 hours.

17. Beef stir·fry

Ingredient:

• 1 lb flank steak or sirloin, thinly sliced against the grain
• 2 tbsp vegetable oil
• 1 red bell pepper, sliced
• 1 cup broccoli florets
• 1 cup sliced mushrooms
• 3 cloves garlic, minced
• 1 tbsp grated fresh ginger
• 2 tbsp soy sauce
• 1 tbsp rice vinegar
• 1 tsp sesame oil
• Salt and pepper to taste
• Cooked rice, for serving

Instructions:

1. In a large skillet or wok, heat the vegetable oil over high heat.

2. Add the sliced beef and stir·fry for 2·3 minutes, until the beef is lightly browned. Remove the beef from the pan and set aside.

3. Add the bell pepper, broccoli, and mushrooms to the hot pan. Stir·fry for 3·4 minutes, until the vegetables are crisp·tender.

4. Push the vegetables to the side of the pan and add the garlic and ginger. Cook for 1 minute, until fragrant.

5. Return the beef to the pan and add the soy sauce, rice vinegar, and sesame oil. Toss everything together and cook for 2·3 minutes, until the beef is cooked through and the sauce has thickened slightly.

6. Season with salt and pepper to taste.

7. Serve the beef stir·fry immediately over steamed rice.

Tips:
• Slice the beef against the grain for the most tender texture.
• Use a high·heat oil like vegetable, canola, or peanut oil for stir·frying.
• Adjust the cooking time for the vegetables based on their firmness • harder veggies like broccoli may need a bit longer.

18. Chicken fajitas

Ingredient:

• 1 lb boneless, skinless chicken breasts, sliced into thin strips
• 2 tbsp olive oil
• 1 packet fajita seasoning
• 1 red bell pepper, sliced
• 1 green bell pepper, sliced
• 1 onion, sliced
• 8•10 flour tortillas
• Toppings: shredded lettuce, diced tomatoes, shredded cheese, sour cream, salsa

Instructions:

1. In a large skillet or wok, heat the olive oil over medium•high heat.

2. Add the sliced chicken and fajita seasoning. Stir•fry for 5•7 minutes, until the chicken is cooked through.

3. Add the sliced bell peppers and onion to the skillet. Continue stir•frying for 3•4 minutes, until the vegetables are tender•crisp.

4. Remove the skillet from heat and keep the chicken and vegetables warm.

5. Warm the flour tortillas according to package instructions.

6. To assemble the fajitas, place some of the chicken and vegetable mixture onto a warm tortilla. Top with your desired toppings such as shredded lettuce, diced tomatoes, shredded cheese, sour cream, and salsa.

7. Fold the tortilla over the filling and serve immediately.

Tips:
• Use a variety of bell peppers for more color and flavor.
• Marinate the chicken in the fajita seasoning and a bit of lime juice for extra flavor.
• Grill the chicken and vegetables for a smoky, charred flavor.
• Serve the fajita fillings and toppings in separate bowls so everyone can customize their own.
• Warm the tortillas in a dry skillet or wrap in foil and heat in the oven for best results.
• Leftovers can be stored in the refrigerator for up to 3 days.

19. Beef and broccoli

Ingredient:

• 1 lb flank steak, thinly sliced against the grain
• 2 tbsp vegetable oil
• 3 cups broccoli florets
• 3 cloves garlic, minced
• 1 tbsp grated fresh ginger
• 2 tbsp soy sauce
• 1 tbsp rice vinegar
• 1 tsp sesame oil
• 1/4 tsp red pepper flakes (optional)
• Salt and pepper to taste
• Cooked rice, for serving

Instructions:

1. In a large skillet or wok, heat the vegetable oil over high heat.

2. Add the sliced beef and stir•fry for 2•3 minutes, until the beef is lightly browned. Remove the beef from the pan and set aside.

3. Add the broccoli florets to the hot pan and stir•fry for 3•4 minutes, until the broccoli is crisp•tender.

4. Push the broccoli to the side of the pan and add the garlic and ginger. Cook for 1 minute, until fragrant.

5. Return the beef to the pan and add the soy sauce, rice vinegar, sesame oil, and red pepper flakes (if using). Toss everything together and cook for 2•3 minutes, until the beef is cooked through and the sauce has thickened slightly.

6. Season with salt and pepper to taste. Serve the beef and broccoli immediately over steamed rice.

Tips:
• Slice the beef against the grain for the most tender texture.
• Use a high•heat oil like vegetable, canola, or peanut oil for stir•frying.
• Adjust the cooking time for the broccoli based on how crisp you like it.
• Feel free to add other vegetables like mushrooms, snow peas, or carrots.
• Add a splash of water or broth if the stir•fry seems too dry.

20. Chicken teriyaki

Ingredient:

• 1 lb boneless, skinless chicken breasts, cut into 1•inch pieces
• 1/2 cup soy sauce
• 1/4 cup brown sugar
• 2 tbsp rice vinegar
• 2 tbsp sesame oil
• 2 cloves garlic, minced
• 1 tsp grated fresh ginger
• 1/4 tsp red pepper flakes (optional)
• 2 tbsp cornstarch
• 2 tbsp water
• Cooked rice, for serving
• Sesame seeds and sliced green onions, for garnish

Instructions:

1. In a large resealable bag or bowl, combine the soy sauce, brown sugar, rice vinegar, sesame oil, garlic, ginger, and red pepper flakes (if using). Add the chicken and toss to coat. Marinate for at least 30 minutes, or up to 4 hours in the refrigerator.

2. In a small bowl, whisk together the cornstarch and water to make a slurry. Set aside.

3. Heat a large skillet or wok over medium•high heat. Remove the chicken from the marinade and add it to the hot pan. Cook for 5•7 minutes, stirring occasionally, until the chicken is cooked through.

4. Pour the reserved marinade into the pan and bring to a simmer. Stir in the cornstarch slurry and cook for 1•2 minutes, until the sauce has thickened.

5. Serve the chicken teriyaki immediately over steamed rice, garnished with sesame seeds and sliced green onions.

Tips:
• Use fresh, high•quality soy sauce and rice vinegar for the best flavor.
• Marinate the chicken for at least 30 minutes, but up to 4 hours, for maximum flavor.
• Adjust the amount of red pepper flakes to control the heat level.
• Serve with steamed broccoli or other vegetables for a complete meal.
• Leftovers can be stored in the refrigerator for up to 4 days.

21. Beef tacos

Ingredient:

- 1 lb ground beef
- 1 packet taco seasoning
- 1/2 cup water
- 8•10 taco shells or soft tortillas
- Shredded lettuce
- Diced tomatoes
- Shredded cheddar cheese
- Sour cream (optional)
- Salsa (optional)

Instructions:

1. In a large skillet over medium•high heat, cook the ground beef until browned and crumbled, 5•7 minutes. Drain any excess fat.

2. Stir in the taco seasoning and water. Bring to a simmer and cook for 2•3 minutes, until the sauce has thickened.

3. Warm the taco shells or tortillas according to package instructions.

4. To assemble the tacos, layer each shell or tortilla with some of the seasoned ground beef, shredded lettuce, diced tomatoes, and shredded cheddar cheese.

5. Top with a dollop of sour cream and/or salsa, if desired.

6. Serve the beef tacos immediately and enjoy!

Tips:
- Use a blend of ground beef and ground turkey for a leaner taco filling.
- Add diced onions, jalapeños, or other veggies to the beef mixture for extra flavor.
- For a creamier taco, mix the ground beef with a bit of sour cream or cream cheese.
- Serve the taco fillings and toppings in separate bowls so everyone can customize their own.
- Leftovers can be stored in the refrigerator for up to 3 days.

22. Chicken Caesar salad

Ingredient:

• 2 boneless, skinless chicken breasts
• 1 tbsp olive oil
• 1 tsp garlic powder
• Salt and pepper to taste
• 8 cups chopped romaine lettuce
• 1 cup croutons
• 1/2 cup grated Parmesan cheese
• Caesar dressing (store•bought or homemade)

For the Homemade Caesar Dressing:

• 1/2 cup mayonnaise
• 2 tbsp lemon juice
• 2 tbsp Dijon mustard
• 2 cloves garlic, minced
• 1 tsp Worcestershire sauce
• 1/4 cup grated Parmesan cheese
• Salt and pepper to taste

Instructions:

1. Preheat oven to 400°F. Season the chicken breasts with garlic powder, salt, and pepper.

2. Heat the olive oil in a large oven•safe skillet over medium•high heat. Add the chicken and sear for 2•3 minutes per side until golden brown.

3. Transfer the skillet to the preheated oven and bake for 15•20 minutes, until the chicken is cooked through. Allow to cool slightly, then slice or shred the chicken.

4. If making the homemade Caesar dressing, whisk together all the dressing ingredients in a small bowl until well combined.

5. In a large salad bowl, combine the chopped romaine lettuce, sliced or shredded chicken, croutons, and Parmesan cheese.

6. Drizzle the Caesar dressing over the salad and toss gently to coat.

7. Serve the chicken Caesar salad immediately.

23. Beef and cheese quesadillas

Ingredient:

- 1 lb ground beef
- 1 packet taco seasoning
- 1/2 cup water
- 8 flour tortillas (8•inch size)
- 2 cups shredded cheddar or Monterey Jack cheese
- Salsa, sour cream, and guacamole for serving (optional)

Instructions:

1. In a large skillet over medium•high heat, cook the ground beef until browned and crumbled, 5•7 minutes. Drain any excess fat.

2. Stir in the taco seasoning and water. Bring to a simmer and cook for 2•3 minutes, until the sauce has thickened. Remove from heat and set aside.

3. Preheat a large skillet or griddle over medium heat.

4. Place one tortilla in the hot pan. On one half of the tortilla, layer some of the seasoned ground beef and shredded cheese.

5. Fold the other half of the tortilla over the filled half to create a half•moon shape.

6. Cook the quesadilla for 2•3 minutes per side, until the tortilla is lightly browned and the cheese is melted.

7. Repeat the process with the remaining tortillas, beef, and cheese to make 4 total quesadillas.

8. Cut each quesadilla in half and serve warm, with salsa, sour cream, and guacamole on the side for dipping, if desired.

Tips:
- Use a blend of cheeses, such as cheddar and Monterey Jack, for more flavor.
- Add diced onions, bell peppers, or jalapeños to the beef mixture for extra flavor.
- Brush the outside of the tortillas with a little oil or melted butter for extra crispiness.
- Keep the cooked quesadillas warm in a 200°F oven while you cook the remaining ones.
- Leftovers can be reheated in a skillet or the microwave.

24. Chicken and vegetable stir·fry

Ingredient:

- 1 lb boneless, skinless chicken breasts, cut into 1·inch pieces
- 2 tbsp vegetable oil
- 1 cup broccoli florets
- 1 red bell pepper, sliced
- 1 cup sliced mushrooms
- 1 cup snow peas or snap peas
- 3 cloves garlic, minced
- 1 tbsp grated fresh ginger
- 2 tbsp soy sauce
- 1 tbsp rice vinegar
- 1 tsp sesame oil
- Salt and pepper to taste
- Cooked rice, for serving

Instructions:

1. Heat the vegetable oil in a large skillet or wok over high heat.

2. Add the chicken and stir·fry for 3·4 minutes, until lightly browned. Remove the chicken from the pan and set aside.

3. Add the broccoli, bell pepper, mushrooms, and snow peas to the hot pan. Stir·fry for 3·4 minutes, until the vegetables are crisp·tender.

4. Push the vegetables to the side of the pan and add the garlic and ginger. Cook for 1 minute, until fragrant.

5. Return the chicken to the pan and add the soy sauce, rice vinegar, and sesame oil. Toss everything together and cook for 2·3 minutes, until the chicken is cooked through and the sauce has thickened slightly.

6. Season with salt and pepper to taste. Serve the chicken and vegetable stir·fry immediately over steamed rice.

Tips:
- Use a variety of fresh, crisp vegetables for the best texture.
- Adjust the cooking time for the vegetables based on their firmness · harder veggies like broccoli may need a bit longer.

25. Beef and bean burritos

Ingredient:

- 1 lb ground beef
- 1 packet taco seasoning
- 1 (15 oz) can refried beans
- 8 large flour tortillas
- 1 cup shredded cheddar cheese
- Salsa, sour cream, and guacamole for serving (optional)

Instructions:

1. In a large skillet over medium•high heat, cook the ground beef until browned and crumbled, 5•7 minutes. Drain any excess fat.

2. Stir in the taco seasoning and the amount of water called for on the seasoning packet. Bring to a simmer and cook for 2•3 minutes, until the sauce has thickened. Remove from heat.

3. Warm the refried beans in a small saucepan or in the microwave until heated through.

4. Lay the flour tortillas on a flat surface. Spread about 2•3 tablespoons of refried beans down the center of each tortilla.

5. Top the beans with a few spoonfuls of the seasoned ground beef.

6. Sprinkle the shredded cheddar cheese over the beef.

7. Fold the bottom of the tortilla up over the filling, then fold in the sides and continue rolling up tightly to create a burrito.

8. Heat a large skillet or griddle over medium heat. Place the burritos seam•side down in the hot pan and cook for 2•3 minutes per side, until lightly browned.

9. Serve the beef and bean burritos warm, with salsa, sour cream, and guacamole on the side for dipping, if desired.

Tips:
- Use pinto or black beans for the refried beans.
- Add diced onions, bell peppers, or jalapeños to the beef mixture for extra flavor.

26. Chicken and rice casserole

Ingredient:

• 1 lb boneless, skinless chicken breasts, cubed
• 1 cup uncooked long•grain white rice
• 1 (10.5 oz) can cream of chicken soup
• 1 (10.5 oz) can cream of mushroom soup
• 1 cup milk
• 1 cup frozen peas
• 1/2 cup shredded cheddar cheese
• 1/4 cup sliced almonds (optional)
• Salt and pepper to taste

Instructions:

1. Preheat oven to 375°F. Grease a 9x13 inch baking dish.

2. In a large bowl, combine the cubed chicken, uncooked rice, cream of chicken soup, cream of mushroom soup, milk, and frozen peas. Season with salt and pepper.

3. Transfer the chicken and rice mixture to the prepared baking dish. Spread it out evenly.

4. Cover the dish with foil and bake for 45 minutes.

5. Remove the foil, sprinkle the shredded cheddar cheese and sliced almonds (if using) over the top.

6. Return the casserole to the oven and bake for an additional 15 minutes, or until the rice is tender and the cheese is melted and bubbly.

7. Let the casserole cool for 5•10 minutes before serving.

Tips:
• Use a combination of cream of chicken and cream of mushroom soups for extra flavor.
• Substitute the peas with other frozen vegetables like broccoli or mixed veggies.
• For a creamier texture, use 1 1/2 cups of milk instead of 1 cup.
• Top the casserole with crushed crackers or breadcrumbs for a crispy topping.

27. Beef and mushroom stroganoff

Ingredient:

• 1 lb beef sirloin or tenderloin, cut into 1·inch cubes
• 2 tbsp olive oil
• 8 oz cremini or button mushrooms, sliced
• 1 onion, diced
• 3 cloves garlic, minced
• 2 tbsp all·purpose flour
• 1 cup beef broth
• 1 cup sour cream
• 2 tbsp Dijon mustard
• 1 tsp Worcestershire sauce
• Salt and pepper to taste
• Cooked egg noodles, for serving

Instructions:

1. In a large skillet or Dutch oven, heat the olive oil over medium·high heat. Add the beef cubes and cook for 2·3 minutes per side, until browned on the outside but still pink in the center. Remove the beef from the pan and set aside.

2. Add the sliced mushrooms and diced onion to the same pan. Cook for 5·7 minutes, stirring occasionally, until the mushrooms are tender and the onions are translucent.

3. Add the minced garlic and cook for 1 minute, until fragrant.

4. Sprinkle the flour over the mushroom mixture and stir to coat. Cook for 1 minute.

5. Gradually whisk in the beef broth, scraping up any browned bits from the bottom of the pan. Bring the mixture to a simmer and cook for 2·3 minutes, until the sauce has thickened.

6. Reduce the heat to low and stir in the sour cream, Dijon mustard, and Worcestershire sauce. Season with salt and pepper to taste.

7. Return the seared beef and any accumulated juices to the pan. Gently stir to combine. Serve the beef and mushroom stroganoff immediately over cooked egg noodles.

Tips:
• Use a tender cut of beef like sirloin or tenderloin for the best texture.
• Sear the beef in batches to get a nice brown crust.

28. Chicken and broccoli Alfredo

Ingredient:

• 8 oz fettuccine pasta
• 1 lb boneless, skinless chicken breasts, cut into 1•inch pieces
• 2 tbsp olive oil
• 1/2 tsp salt
• 1/4 tsp black pepper
• 2 cups broccoli florets
• 2 cups heavy cream
• 1 cup grated Parmesan cheese
• 2 cloves garlic, minced
• 2 tbsp unsalted butter
• 2 tbsp chopped fresh parsley (optional)

Instructions:

1. Bring a large pot of salted water to a boil. Add the fettuccine and cook according to package instructions until al dente. Drain and set aside.

2. Season the chicken pieces with salt and pepper. Heat the olive oil in a large skillet over medium•high heat. Add the chicken and cook for 5•7 minutes, until cooked through. Remove the chicken from the skillet and set aside.

3. In the same skillet, add the broccoli florets and a splash of water. Cover and steam the broccoli for 3•4 minutes, until crisp•tender. Remove the broccoli from the skillet and set aside.

4. Reduce the heat to medium and add the heavy cream, Parmesan, and garlic to the skillet. Bring to a simmer and cook for 2•3 minutes, stirring frequently, until the sauce thickens slightly.

5. Reduce the heat to low and stir in the butter until melted and fully incorporated.

6. Add the cooked fettuccine, chicken, and broccoli to the Alfredo sauce and toss to coat everything evenly.

7. Serve immediately, garnished with chopped fresh parsley if desired.

Tips:
• Use boneless, skinless chicken thighs for extra juicy and flavorful chicken.
• For a creamier sauce, use half•and•half or a combination of heavy cream and milk.

29. Beef and potato stew

Ingredient:

- 2 lbs beef stew meat, cut into 1•inch cubes
- 2 tbsp olive oil
- 1 onion, diced
- 3 cloves garlic, minced
- 2 carrots, peeled and diced
- 2 celery stalks, diced
- 2 lbs Yukon Gold potatoes, peeled and diced
- 4 cups beef broth
- 1 cup red wine
- 2 bay leaves
- 2 sprigs fresh thyme
- 1 tsp dried oregano
- Salt and pepper to taste
- Chopped parsley for garnish

Instructions:

1. In a large Dutch oven or heavy bottomed pot, heat the olive oil over medium•high heat. Working in batches if needed, brown the beef cubes on all sides, about 3•4 minutes per batch. Remove beef to a plate.

2. Reduce heat to medium and add the onion, garlic, carrots and celery to the pot. Cook for 5•7 minutes, stirring occasionally, until the vegetables are softened.

3. Pour in the red wine and use a wooden spoon to scrape up any browned bits from the bottom of the pot. Let the wine simmer for 2•3 minutes.

4. Add the browned beef back to the pot along with the potatoes, beef broth, bay leaves, thyme and oregano. Season with salt and pepper.

5. Bring the stew to a boil, then reduce heat to low, cover and simmer for 1.5•2 hours, until the beef is very tender.

6. Remove the bay leaves and thyme sprigs. Taste and adjust seasoning as needed. Serve the beef and potato stew hot, garnished with chopped parsley. Enjoy with crusty bread.

The tender beef, hearty potatoes, and rich broth make this stew so comforting and satisfying. It's the perfect meal for a chilly day.

30. Chicken and spinach lasagna

Ingredient:

• 9 lasagna noodles
• 2 tbsp olive oil
• 1 lb boneless, skinless chicken breasts, diced
• 1 onion, diced
• 3 cloves garlic, minced
• 10 oz frozen chopped spinach, thawed and drained
• 1 (15 oz) container ricotta cheese
• 2 cups shredded mozzarella cheese, divided
• 1/2 cup grated Parmesan cheese
• 1 egg
• 1 tsp dried basil
• 1/2 tsp dried oregano
• Salt and pepper to taste
• 1 (24 oz) jar marinara sauce

Instructions:

1. Preheat oven to 375°F. Cook the lasagna noodles according to package instructions. Drain and set aside.

2. In a large skillet, heat the olive oil over medium•high heat. Add the diced chicken and cook for 5•7 minutes until no longer pink. Remove chicken to a plate.

3. Add the onion to the skillet and cook for 3•4 minutes until softened. Add the garlic and cook for 1 minute more.

4. In a large bowl, mix together the ricotta, 1 cup of the mozzarella, Parmesan, egg, basil, oregano, salt and pepper. Stir in the cooked chicken, onion/garlic mixture, and drained spinach.

5. Spread 1 cup of the marinara sauce in the bottom of a 9x13 inch baking dish. Arrange 3 lasagna noodles over the sauce. Spread half of the chicken•ricotta mixture over the noodles. Top with another 1 cup of sauce.

6. Repeat the layers of noodles, chicken•ricotta mixture and sauce. Top with the remaining 3 noodles and the remaining sauce. Sprinkle the top with the remaining 1 cup of mozzarella cheese.

7. Cover with foil and bake for 40 minutes. Remove foil and bake for 10•15 minutes more, until cheese is melted and lightly browned. Let stand for 10 minutes before serving.

31. Beef and vegetable stir·fry

Ingredient:

- 1 lb beef sirloin or flank steak, thinly sliced
- 2 tbsp vegetable oil
- 3 cloves garlic, minced
- 1 tbsp grated fresh ginger
- 1 red bell pepper, sliced
- 1 cup broccoli florets
- 1 cup sliced mushrooms
- 1 cup snow peas or snap peas
- 2 green onions, sliced
- 2 tbsp soy sauce
- 1 tbsp rice vinegar
- 1 tsp sesame oil
- Salt and pepper to taste
- Cooked rice, for serving

For the Sauce:
- 2 tbsp soy sauce
- 2 tbsp rice vinegar
- 1 tbsp brown sugar
- 1 tsp cornstarch
- 1/4 tsp red pepper flakes (optional)

Instructions:

1. In a small bowl, whisk together all the sauce ingredients and set aside.

2. Heat the vegetable oil in a large skillet or wok over high heat. Add the beef and stir·fry for 2·3 minutes until browned. Remove beef to a plate.

3. Add the garlic and ginger to the skillet and cook for 1 minute until fragrant.

4. Add the bell pepper, broccoli, mushrooms and snow peas. Stir·fry for 3·4 minutes until vegetables are crisp·tender.

5. Return the beef and any juices to the skillet. Pour in the sauce and toss everything together, cooking for 2·3 minutes until the sauce thickens.

6. Remove from heat and stir in the green onions and sesame oil. Season with salt and pepper. Serve the beef and vegetable stir·fry immediately over steamed rice.

32. Chicken and mushroom risotto

Ingredient:

• 4 cups chicken broth
• 2 tbsp olive oil
• 8 oz cremini or button mushrooms, sliced
• 1 onion, diced
• 2 cloves garlic, minced
• 1 1/2 cups arborio rice
• 1/2 cup dry white wine
• 2 cups cooked, shredded chicken
• 1/2 cup grated Parmesan cheese
• 2 tbsp butter
• Salt and pepper to taste
• Chopped parsley for garnish

Instructions:

1. In a saucepan, bring the chicken broth to a simmer and keep it warm over low heat.

2. In a large skillet, heat the olive oil over medium•high heat. Add the mushrooms and cook for 5•7 minutes until browned. Remove the mushrooms to a plate.

3. Reduce the heat to medium and add the onion to the skillet. Cook for 3•4 minutes until softened. Add the garlic and cook for 1 minute more.

4. Add the arborio rice to the skillet and stir to coat with the oil. Cook for 2•3 minutes until the rice is lightly toasted.

5. Pour in the white wine and cook, stirring constantly, until the wine is absorbed, about 2 minutes.

6. Begin adding the warm chicken broth, 1/2 cup at a time, stirring constantly until each addition is absorbed before adding more. This will take 18•22 minutes total.

7. Once all the broth has been added and the rice is tender, stir in the cooked chicken, Parmesan, butter, and the sautéed mushrooms. Season with salt and pepper. Serve the risotto immediately, garnished with chopped parsley.

The creamy, cheesy risotto paired with tender chicken and earthy mushrooms makes this a truly comforting and satisfying dish.

33. Beef and black bean chili

Ingredient:

- 2 lbs ground beef
- 1 onion, diced
- 3 cloves garlic, minced
- 2 tbsp chili powder
- 1 tbsp ground cumin
- 1 tsp dried oregano
- 1 tsp smoked paprika
- 1/2 tsp cayenne pepper (or to taste)
- 1 (15 oz) can black beans, drained and rinsed
- 1 (15 oz) can diced tomatoes
- 1 (6 oz) can tomato paste
- 2 cups beef broth
- Salt and pepper to taste
- Toppings: shredded cheddar, sour cream, chopped onions, etc.

Instructions:

1. In a large pot or Dutch oven, cook the ground beef over medium•high heat, breaking it up with a wooden spoon, until browned and cooked through, about 5•7 minutes. Drain excess fat.

2. Add the diced onion and garlic to the pot. Cook for 3•4 minutes until the onion is translucent.

3. Stir in the chili powder, cumin, oregano, smoked paprika and cayenne. Cook for 1 minute to toast the spices.

4. Pour in the black beans, diced tomatoes, tomato paste and beef broth. Stir to combine.

5. Bring the chili to a simmer, then reduce heat to medium•low. Let the chili simmer for 30•40 minutes, stirring occasionally, until thickened.

6. Taste and season with salt and pepper as needed.

7. Serve the beef and black bean chili hot, topped with shredded cheddar, sour cream, chopped onions, or any other desired toppings.

The blend of spices, tender beef, and hearty black beans makes this chili so flavorful and satisfying. Adjust the heat level by adding more or less cayenne pepper.

34. Chicken and corn chowder

Ingredient:

• 2 tbsp olive oil
• 1 onion, diced
• 2 carrots, peeled and diced
• 2 celery stalks, diced
• 3 cloves garlic, minced
• 4 cups chicken broth
• 2 cups diced cooked chicken
• 2 cups frozen corn kernels
• 2 medium potatoes, peeled and diced
• 1 tsp dried thyme
• 1 bay leaf
• Salt and pepper to taste
• 1 cup half and half or heavy cream (optional)

Instructions:

1. In a large pot or Dutch oven, heat the olive oil over medium heat. Add the onion, carrots, celery and garlic. Cook for 5•7 minutes until the vegetables are softened.

2. Pour in the chicken broth and add the diced chicken, corn, potatoes, thyme and bay leaf. Season with salt and pepper.

3. Bring the chowder to a simmer and cook for 20•25 minutes, until the potatoes are tender.

4. If using, stir in the half and half or cream and heat through, but do not boil.

5. Remove the bay leaf. Taste and adjust seasoning as needed.

6. Serve the chowder hot, garnished with chopped parsley or chives if desired. Enjoy!

The creamy broth, tender chicken, and sweet corn make this chowder so comforting and delicious. It's perfect for a cozy meal on a chilly day.

35. Beef and barley soup

Ingredient:

- 2 lbs beef stew meat, cut into 1•inch cubes
- 2 tbsp olive oil
- 1 onion, diced
- 3 carrots, peeled and diced
- 3 celery stalks, diced
- 4 cloves garlic, minced
- 8 cups beef broth
- 1 cup pearl barley
- 1 (14.5 oz) can diced tomatoes
- 2 bay leaves
- 1 tsp dried thyme
- Salt and pepper to taste
- Chopped parsley for garnish

Instructions:

1. In a large pot or Dutch oven, heat the olive oil over medium•high heat. Working in batches if needed, brown the beef cubes on all sides, about 3•4 minutes per batch. Remove beef to a plate.

2. Reduce heat to medium and add the onion, carrots, celery and garlic to the pot. Cook for 5•7 minutes, stirring occasionally, until the vegetables are softened.

3. Pour in the beef broth and add the browned beef, pearl barley, diced tomatoes, bay leaves and thyme. Season with salt and pepper.

4. Bring the soup to a boil, then reduce heat to low, cover and simmer for 1•1.5 hours, until the beef is very tender and the barley is cooked through.

5. Remove the bay leaves. Taste and adjust seasoning as needed.

6. Serve the beef and barley soup hot, garnished with chopped parsley. Enjoy with crusty bread.

The tender beef, chewy barley, and hearty vegetables make this soup so comforting and satisfying. The long simmer allows the flavors to meld together beautifully.

36. Chicken and sweet potato curry

Ingredient:

• 1 lb boneless, skinless chicken thighs, cut into 1•inch pieces
• 2 tbsp olive oil
• 1 onion, diced
• 3 cloves garlic, minced
• 1 tbsp grated fresh ginger
• 2 tsp curry powder
• 1 tsp ground cumin
• 1 tsp ground coriander
• 1/4 tsp cayenne pepper (or to taste)
• 1 (14 oz) can coconut milk
• 1 lb sweet potatoes, peeled and diced
• 1 cup chicken broth
• 1 cup frozen peas
• Salt and pepper to taste
• Chopped cilantro for garnish
• Cooked basmati rice, for serving

Instructions:

1. In a large skillet or Dutch oven, heat the olive oil over medium•high heat. Add the chicken and cook for 3•4 minutes until lightly browned. Remove chicken to a plate.

2. Reduce heat to medium and add the onion to the skillet. Cook for 5 minutes until softened. Add the garlic and ginger and cook for 1 minute more.

3. Stir in the curry powder, cumin, coriander and cayenne. Cook for 1 minute to toast the spices.

4. Pour in the coconut milk and chicken broth. Add the diced sweet potatoes and return the chicken to the pot.

5. Bring the curry to a simmer, then reduce heat to medium•low. Cover and cook for 20•25 minutes, until the sweet potatoes are tender.

6. Stir in the frozen peas and cook for 5 minutes more. Season with salt and pepper to taste. Serve the chicken and sweet potato curry over steamed basmati rice, garnished with chopped cilantro.

The creamy coconut milk, aromatic spices, and tender chicken and sweet potatoes make this curry so flavorful and comforting. Adjust the heat level with more or less cayenne.

37. Beef and vegetable curry

Ingredient:

- 1 lb beef stew meat, cut into 1•inch cubes
- 2 tbsp vegetable oil
- 1 onion, diced
- 3 cloves garlic, minced
- 1 tbsp grated fresh ginger
- 2 tsp curry powder
- 1 tsp ground cumin
- 1 tsp ground coriander
- 1/2 tsp cayenne pepper (or to taste)
- 1 cup beef broth
- 1 (14oz) can diced tomatoes
- 1 medium potato, peeled and diced
- 1 cup cauliflower florets
- 1 cup frozen peas
- 1 cup coconut milk
- Salt and pepper to taste
- Chopped cilantro for garnish

Instructions:

1. In a large pot or Dutch oven, heat the vegetable oil over medium•high heat. Add the beef cubes and brown on all sides, about 5 minutes total. Remove beef to a plate.

2. Reduce heat to medium and add the onion to the pot. Cook for 3•4 minutes until softened. Add the garlic and ginger and cook for 1 minute more.

3. Stir in the curry powder, cumin, coriander and cayenne. Cook for 1 minute to toast the spices.

4. Pour in the beef broth and diced tomatoes. Add the potatoes, cauliflower and peas. Bring to a simmer.

5. Return the browned beef and any juices to the pot. Reduce heat to medium•low and simmer for 30•40 minutes, until beef is very tender.

6. Stir in the coconut milk and season with salt and pepper to taste. Serve the curry over basmati rice, garnished with chopped cilantro.

The blend of aromatic spices, tender beef, and fresh vegetables makes this curry so flavorful and comforting. Adjust the heat level to your preference.

38. Chicken and vegetable kebabs

Ingredient:

• 1 lb boneless, skinless chicken breasts, cut into 1•inch cubes
• 1 red bell pepper, cut into 1•inch pieces
• 1 yellow bell pepper, cut into 1•inch pieces
• 1 red onion, cut into 1•inch pieces
• 8 oz mushrooms, halved
• 1 zucchini, cut into 1•inch pieces
• 2 tbsp olive oil
• 2 tbsp lemon juice
• 2 tsp dried oregano
• 1 tsp garlic powder
• Salt and pepper to taste
• Wooden or metal skewers

For the Marinade:
• 1/4 cup olive oil
• 2 tbsp lemon juice
• 2 cloves garlic, minced
• 1 tsp dried oregano
• 1/2 tsp salt
• 1/4 tsp black pepper

Instructions:

1. In a large bowl, whisk together the marinade ingredients. Add the chicken cubes and toss to coat. Cover and refrigerate for 30 minutes to 1 hour.

2. In a separate bowl, toss the chopped vegetables with the 2 tbsp olive oil, 2 tbsp lemon juice, 2 tsp oregano, garlic powder, salt and pepper.

3. Preheat grill or grill pan to medium•high heat.

4. Thread the marinated chicken and seasoned vegetables onto skewers, alternating the ingredients.

5. Grill the kebabs for 12•15 minutes, turning occasionally, until the chicken is cooked through and the vegetables are tender.

6. Serve the chicken and vegetable kebabs immediately, with any extra marinade drizzled over the top.

These colorful and flavorful kebabs are perfect for grilling. The marinade keeps the chicken juicy and the vegetables add a nice crunch. Serve with rice or pita bread for a complete meal.

39. Beef and cheese enchiladas

Ingredient:

- 1 lb ground beef
- 1 onion, diced
- 3 cloves garlic, minced
- 2 tbsp chili powder
- 1 tsp ground cumin
- 1 tsp dried oregano
- Salt and pepper to taste
- 12 corn tortillas
- 2 cups shredded cheddar cheese
- 1 (15 oz) can enchilada sauce

For the Sauce:

- 2 tbsp olive oil
- 2 tbsp all·purpose flour
- 2 cups chicken or beef broth
- 1 (4 oz) can diced green chiles
- 1 tsp chili powder
- 1/2 tsp ground cumin
- Salt and pepper to taste

Instructions:

1. Preheat oven to 350°F. Grease a 9x13 inch baking dish.

2. In a large skillet, cook the ground beef over medium·high heat, breaking it up with a wooden spoon, until browned and cooked through, about 5·7 minutes. Drain excess fat.

3. Add the diced onion and garlic to the skillet. Cook for 3·4 minutes until the onion is translucent.

4. Stir in the chili powder, cumin, oregano, salt and pepper. Cook for 1 minute.

5. To make the sauce, heat the olive oil in a saucepan over medium heat. Whisk in the flour and cook for 1 minute. Gradually whisk in the broth and bring to a simmer. Stir in the green chiles, chili powder, cumin, salt and pepper. Simmer for 5 minutes until thickened.

6. Spread 1/2 cup of the enchilada sauce in the bottom of the prepared baking dish.

7. Warm the tortillas according to package instructions. Spoon about 2·3 tbsp of the beef mixture down the center of each tortilla. Roll up tightly and place seam·side down in the baking dish.

8. Pour the remaining enchilada sauce over the rolled enchiladas and sprinkle with the shredded cheddar cheese. Bake for 20·25 minutes, until the cheese is melted and bubbly. Serve the beef and cheese enchiladas hot, garnished with chopped onions, cilantro, sour cream, etc.

The seasoned ground beef, melty cheese, and homemade enchilada sauce make these enchiladas so flavorful and satisfying.

40. Chicken and avocado wraps

Ingredient:

• 2 cups cooked, shredded chicken
• 1 avocado, diced
• 1/4 cup diced red onion
• 1/4 cup chopped cilantro
• Juice of 1 lime
• 1 tbsp olive oil
• Salt and pepper to taste
• 4•6 large tortilla or wrap shells

For the Dressing:
• 1/4 cup plain Greek yogurt
• 2 tbsp mayonnaise
• 1 tbsp Dijon mustard
• 1 tbsp honey
• 1 tbsp water
• Salt and pepper to taste

Instructions:

1. In a medium bowl, combine the shredded chicken, diced avocado, red onion, cilantro, lime juice and olive oil. Season with salt and pepper and mix well.

2. In a small bowl, whisk together all the dressing ingredients until smooth and creamy. Season with salt and pepper.

3. Lay the tortilla or wrap shells out on a flat surface. Divide the chicken and avocado mixture evenly among the wraps, spooning it down the center.

4. Drizzle the dressing over the filling.

5. Fold the bottom of the wrap up over the filling, then fold in the sides and continue rolling up tightly into a wrap.

6. Slice the wraps in half diagonally and serve immediately.

The creamy avocado, tangy dressing, and tender chicken make these wraps so flavorful and satisfying. They're perfect for a quick and healthy lunch or light dinner.

41. Beef and vegetable stir·fry

Ingredient:

- 3 cloves garlic, minced
- 1 tbsp grated fresh ginger
- 1/4 cup beef broth
- 2 tbsp brown sugar
- 1 tbsp rice vinegar
- 1 tsp sesame oil
- Salt and pepper to taste
- Cooked rice, for serving

- 1 lb flank steak, thinly sliced against the grain
- 2 tbsp soy sauce, divided
- 2 tsp cornstarch, divided
- 2 tbsp vegetable oil, divided
- 1 red bell pepper, sliced
- 1 cup broccoli florets
- 1 cup sliced mushrooms

Instructions:

1. In a medium bowl, toss the sliced beef with 1 tbsp soy sauce and 1 tsp cornstarch. Let marinate for 15 minutes.

2. Heat 1 tbsp of the vegetable oil in a large skillet or wok over high heat. Add the beef in a single layer and cook undisturbed for 1·2 minutes to get a nice sear. Flip and cook for 1 minute more. Remove beef to a plate.

3. Add the remaining 1 tbsp oil to the skillet. Add the bell pepper, broccoli and mushrooms and stir·fry for 3·4 minutes until crisp·tender.

4. Push the vegetables to the sides of the skillet. Add the garlic and ginger to the center and cook for 1 minute until fragrant.

5. In a small bowl, whisk together the beef broth, brown sugar, rice vinegar, remaining 1 tbsp soy sauce, and remaining 1 tsp cornstarch.

6. Pour the sauce mixture into the skillet and bring to a simmer. Cook for 1·2 minutes until thickened slightly.

7. Return the seared beef and any juices to the skillet. Toss everything together and cook for 2·3 minutes more until the beef is cooked through.

8. Remove from heat and stir in the sesame oil. Season with salt and pepper to taste. Serve the beef and vegetable stir·fry immediately over steamed rice.

The tender beef, crisp vegetables, and savory·sweet sauce make this stir·fry so flavorful and satisfying. Adjust the heat with more or less red pepper flakes.

42. Chicken and black bean burritos

Ingredient:

- 1 lb boneless, skinless chicken breasts, diced
- 1 tbsp olive oil
- 1 onion, diced
- 3 cloves garlic, minced
- 1 tbsp chili powder
- 1 tsp ground cumin
- 1 (15 oz) can black beans, drained and rinsed
- 1 cup cooked rice
- 1 cup shredded cheddar or Monterey Jack cheese
- 8•10 large flour tortillas
- Toppings: salsa, sour cream, shredded lettuce, etc.

For the Sauce:
- 2 tbsp olive oil
- 2 tbsp all•purpose flour
- 2 cups chicken or vegetable broth
- 1 (4 oz) can diced green chiles
- 1 tsp chili powder
- 1/2 tsp ground cumin
- Salt and pepper to taste

Instructions:

1. In a large skillet, heat the 1 tbsp olive oil over medium•high heat. Add the diced chicken and cook for 5•7 minutes until no longer pink. Remove chicken to a plate.

2. In the same skillet, sauté the diced onion for 3•4 minutes until softened. Add the minced garlic and cook for 1 minute more.

3. Stir in the chili powder, cumin, black beans and cooked rice. Cook for 2•3 minutes to heat through.

4. Add the cooked chicken back to the skillet and stir to combine. Remove from heat.

5. To make the sauce, heat the 2 tbsp olive oil in a saucepan over medium heat. Whisk in the flour and cook for 1 minute. Gradually whisk in the broth and bring to a simmer. Stir in the green chiles, chili powder, cumin, salt and pepper. Simmer for 5 minutes until thickened.

6. Warm the tortillas according to package instructions. Spoon some of the chicken and black bean mixture down the center of each tortilla. Top with a few tablespoons of the sauce and a sprinkle of shredded cheese.

7. Fold the bottom of the tortilla up over the filling, then fold in the sides and continue rolling up tightly into a burrito.

8. Serve the chicken and black bean burritos warm, with desired toppings like salsa, sour cream and shredded lettuce.

43. Beef and broccoli stir·fry

Ingredient:

- 1 lb flank steak, thinly sliced against the grain
- 2 tbsp soy sauce, divided
- 2 tsp cornstarch, divided
- 2 tbsp vegetable oil, divided
- 3 cups broccoli florets
- 3 cloves garlic, minced
- 1 tbsp grated fresh ginger
- 1/4 cup beef broth
- 2 tbsp brown sugar
- 1 tbsp rice vinegar
- 1 tsp sesame oil
- Salt and pepper to taste
- Cooked rice, for serving

Instructions:

1. In a medium bowl, toss the sliced beef with 1 tbsp soy sauce and 1 tsp cornstarch. Let marinate for 15 minutes.

2. Heat 1 tbsp of the vegetable oil in a large skillet or wok over high heat. Add the beef in a single layer and cook undisturbed for 1·2 minutes to get a nice sear. Flip and cook for 1 minute more. Remove beef to a plate.

3. Add the remaining 1 tbsp oil to the skillet. Add the broccoli florets and stir·fry for 2·3 minutes until crisp·tender.

4. Push the broccoli to the sides of the skillet. Add the garlic and ginger to the center and cook for 1 minute until fragrant.

5. In a small bowl, whisk together the beef broth, brown sugar, rice vinegar, remaining 1 tbsp soy sauce, and remaining 1 tsp cornstarch.

6. Pour the sauce mixture into the skillet and bring to a simmer. Cook for 1·2 minutes until thickened slightly.

7. Return the seared beef and any juices to the skillet. Toss everything together and cook for 2·3 minutes more until the beef is cooked through.

8. Remove from heat and stir in the sesame oil. Season with salt and pepper to taste. Serve the beef and broccoli stir·fry immediately over steamed rice.

44. Chicken and pineapple fried rice

Ingredient:

• 2 cups cooked, diced chicken
• 2 tbsp vegetable oil
• 3 eggs, lightly beaten
• 1 onion, diced
• 3 cloves garlic, minced
• 1 cup diced pineapple
• 3 cups cooked and chilled white rice
• 2 tbsp soy sauce
• 1 tsp sesame oil
• 1/2 tsp ground ginger
• Salt and pepper to taste
• Chopped green onions for garnish

Instructions:

1. Heat 1 tbsp of the vegetable oil in a large skillet or wok over medium•high heat. Pour in the beaten eggs and scramble them, breaking them up into small pieces as they cook. Remove the eggs to a plate.

2. Add the remaining 1 tbsp of oil to the skillet. Add the diced onion and cook for 3•4 minutes until softened.

3. Stir in the minced garlic and cook for 1 minute until fragrant.

4. Add the diced pineapple and cooked chicken to the skillet. Stir and cook for 2•3 minutes.

5. Push the chicken and pineapple mixture to the sides of the skillet. Add the chilled rice to the center and break it up with a spatula. Let the rice fry undisturbed for 2•3 minutes to get a little crispy.

6. Stir the rice together with the chicken and pineapple. Drizzle in the soy sauce, sesame oil and ground ginger. Toss everything together until well combined.

7. Add the scrambled eggs back to the skillet and stir to incorporate. Season the fried rice with salt and pepper to taste. Serve the chicken and pineapple fried rice hot, garnished with chopped green onions.

The sweet pineapple, savory chicken, and crispy rice make this fried rice so flavorful and satisfying. It's a great way to use up leftover rice and chicken.

45. Beef and potato curry

Ingredient:

- 1 lb beef stew meat, cut into 1•inch cubes
- 2 tbsp vegetable oil
- 1 onion, diced
- 3 cloves garlic, minced
- 1 tbsp grated fresh ginger
- 2 tsp garam masala
- 1 tsp ground cumin
- 1 tsp ground coriander
- 1/2 tsp cayenne pepper (or to taste)
- 1 (14 oz) can diced tomatoes
- 1 cup beef broth
- 1 lb Yukon Gold potatoes, peeled and diced
- 1 cup frozen peas
- 1/2 cup heavy cream or coconut milk
- Salt and pepper to taste
- Chopped cilantro for garnish
- Basmati rice, for serving

Instructions:

1. In a large pot or Dutch oven, heat the vegetable oil over medium•high heat. Add the beef cubes and brown on all sides, about 5 minutes total. Remove beef to a plate.

2. Reduce heat to medium and add the diced onion to the pot. Cook for 5•7 minutes until softened. Add the garlic and ginger and cook for 1 minute more.

3. Stir in the garam masala, cumin, coriander and cayenne. Cook for 1 minute to toast the spices.

4. Pour in the diced tomatoes and beef broth. Add the diced potatoes and return the browned beef to the pot.

5. Bring the curry to a simmer, then reduce heat to medium•low. Cover and cook for 30•40 minutes, until the beef is very tender and the potatoes are cooked through.

6. Stir in the frozen peas and heavy cream or coconut milk. Simmer for 5 minutes more.

7. Season the curry with salt and pepper to taste.

8. Serve the beef and potato curry immediately over steamed basmati rice, garnished with chopped cilantro.

The tender beef, hearty potatoes, and aromatic spices make this curry so comforting and flavorful. Adjust the heat with more or less cayenne.

46. Chicken and vegetable curry

Ingredient:

- 1/2 tsp cayenne pepper (or to taste)
- 1 (14 oz) can coconut milk
- 1 cup chicken broth
- 2 medium potatoes, peeled and diced
- 1 cup cauliflower florets
- 1 cup frozen peas
- Salt and pepper to taste
- Chopped cilantro for garnish
- Basmati rice, for serving
- 1 lb boneless, skinless chicken thighs, cut into 1•inch pieces
- 2 tbsp vegetable oil
- 1 onion, diced
- 3 cloves garlic, minced
- 1 tbsp grated fresh ginger
- 2 tsp curry powder
- 1 tsp ground cumin
- 1 tsp ground coriander

Instructions:

1. In a large skillet or Dutch oven, heat the vegetable oil over medium•high heat. Add the chicken pieces and cook for 3•4 minutes until lightly browned. Remove chicken to a plate.

2. Reduce heat to medium and add the diced onion to the skillet. Cook for 5•7 minutes until softened. Add the garlic and ginger and cook for 1 minute more.

3. Stir in the curry powder, cumin, coriander and cayenne. Cook for 1 minute to toast the spices.

4. Pour in the coconut milk and chicken broth. Add the diced potatoes, cauliflower florets and the cooked chicken.

5. Bring the curry to a simmer, then reduce heat to medium•low. Cover and cook for 20•25 minutes, until the potatoes are tender and the chicken is cooked through.

6. Stir in the frozen peas and cook for 5 minutes more. Season with salt and pepper to taste.

7. Serve the chicken and vegetable curry immediately over steamed basmati rice, garnished with chopped cilantro.

The creamy coconut milk, aromatic spices, and tender chicken and vegetables make this curry so flavorful and comforting. Adjust the heat level with more or less cayenne.

47. Beef and cheese quesadillas

Ingredient:

- 1 lb ground beef
- 1 onion, diced
- 2 cloves garlic, minced
- 1 tbsp chili powder
- 1 tsp ground cumin
- 1/2 tsp dried oregano
- Salt and pepper to taste
- 8 large flour tortillas
- 2 cups shredded cheddar or Monterey Jack cheese
- Butter or oil for cooking

Toppings (optional):
- Salsa
- Sour cream
- Guacamole
- Shredded lettuce

Instructions:

1. In a large skillet, cook the ground beef over medium•high heat, breaking it up with a wooden spoon, until browned and cooked through, about 5•7 minutes. Drain excess fat.

2. Add the diced onion and minced garlic to the skillet. Cook for 3•4 minutes until the onion is translucent.

3. Stir in the chili powder, cumin, oregano, salt and pepper. Cook for 1 minute.

4. Remove the beef mixture from the heat and set aside.

5. Heat a large skillet or griddle over medium heat. Lightly butter or oil the surface.

6. Place one tortilla in the skillet. Spread about 1/4 cup of the beef mixture over half of the tortilla. Sprinkle 1/4 cup of the shredded cheese over the beef.

7. Fold the other half of the tortilla over the filling to create a half•moon shape. Cook for 2•3 minutes per side, until the tortilla is lightly browned and the cheese is melted.

8. Repeat with the remaining tortillas, beef and cheese to make 4 quesadillas total.

9. Cut each quesadilla in half and serve warm, with desired toppings like salsa, sour cream and guacamole.

The seasoned ground beef, melty cheese, and crispy tortilla make these quesadillas so satisfying. Adjust the spice level to your preference.

48. Chicken and vegetable stir·fry

Ingredient:

- 1 cup snow peas
- 3 cloves garlic, minced
- 1 tbsp grated fresh ginger
- 1/4 cup chicken broth
- 2 tbsp brown sugar
- 1 tbsp rice vinegar
- 1 tsp sesame oil
- Salt and pepper to taste
- Cooked rice, for serving

- 1 lb boneless, skinless chicken breasts, cut into 1·inch pieces
- 2 tbsp soy sauce, divided
- 2 tsp cornstarch, divided
- 2 tbsp vegetable oil, divided
- 1 red bell pepper, sliced
- 1 cup broccoli florets
- 1 cup sliced mushrooms

Instructions:

1. In a medium bowl, toss the diced chicken with 1 tbsp soy sauce and 1 tsp cornstarch. Let marinate for 15 minutes.

2. Heat 1 tbsp of the vegetable oil in a large skillet or wok over high heat. Add the chicken in a single layer and cook undisturbed for 2·3 minutes to get a nice sear. Flip and cook for 1·2 minutes more. Remove chicken to a plate.

3. Add the remaining 1 tbsp oil to the skillet. Add the bell pepper, broccoli, mushrooms and snow peas. Stir·fry for 3·4 minutes until the vegetables are crisp·tender.

4. Push the vegetables to the sides of the skillet. Add the garlic and ginger to the center and cook for 1 minute until fragrant.

5. In a small bowl, whisk together the chicken broth, brown sugar, rice vinegar, remaining 1 tbsp soy sauce, and remaining 1 tsp cornstarch.

6. Pour the sauce mixture into the skillet and bring to a simmer. Cook for 1·2 minutes until thickened slightly.

7. Return the seared chicken and any juices to the skillet. Toss everything together and cook for 2·3 minutes more until the chicken is cooked through.

8. Remove from heat and stir in the sesame oil. Season with salt and pepper to taste. Serve the chicken and vegetable stir·fry immediately over steamed rice.

The tender chicken, crisp vegetables, and savory·sweet sauce make this stir·fry so flavorful and satisfying. Adjust the heat with more or less red pepper flakes.

49. Beef and bean burritos

Ingredient:

- 1 lb ground beef
- 1 onion, diced
- 3 cloves garlic, minced
- 2 tbsp chili powder
- 1 tsp ground cumin
- 1 tsp dried oregano
- 1 (15 oz) can black beans, drained and rinsed
- 1 (15 oz) can pinto beans, drained and rinsed
- 1 cup shredded cheddar cheese
- 8•10 large flour tortillas
- Toppings: salsa, sour cream, shredded lettuce, etc.

For the Sauce:

- 2 tbsp olive oil
- 2 tbsp all•purpose flour
- 2 cups beef or chicken broth
- 1 (4 oz) can diced green chiles
- 1 tsp chili powder
- 1/2 tsp ground cumin
- Salt and pepper to taste

Instructions:

1. In a large skillet, cook the ground beef over medium•high heat, breaking it up with a wooden spoon, until browned and cooked through, about 5•7 minutes. Drain excess fat.

2. Add the diced onion and garlic to the skillet. Cook for 3•4 minutes until the onion is translucent.

3. Stir in the chili powder, cumin, oregano, salt and pepper. Cook for 1 minute.

4. Add the black beans and pinto beans to the skillet and stir to combine. Remove from heat.

5. To make the sauce, heat the olive oil in a saucepan over medium heat. Whisk in the flour and cook for 1 minute. Gradually whisk in the broth and bring to a simmer. Stir in the green chiles, chili powder, cumin, salt and pepper. Simmer for 5 minutes until thickened.

6. Warm the tortillas according to package instructions. Spoon some of the beef and bean mixture down the center of each tortilla. Top with a few tablespoons of the sauce and a sprinkle of shredded cheddar.

7. Fold the bottom of the tortilla up over the filling, then fold in the sides and continue rolling up tightly into a burrito.

8. Serve the beef and bean burritos warm, with desired toppings like salsa, sour cream and shredded lettuce.

50. Chicken and rice casserole

Ingredient:

• 1 lb boneless, skinless chicken breasts, diced
• 1 cup uncooked long•grain white rice
• 1 (10.5 oz) can cream of chicken soup
• 1 (10.5 oz) can cream of mushroom soup
• 1 cup chicken broth
• 1/2 cup milk
• 1 tsp dried thyme
• 1/2 tsp garlic powder
• Salt and pepper to taste
• 1 cup frozen peas
• 1 cup shredded cheddar cheese

Instructions:

1. Preheat oven to 375°F. Grease a 9x13 inch baking dish.

2. In a large bowl, combine the diced chicken, uncooked rice, cream of chicken soup, cream of mushroom soup, chicken broth, milk, thyme, garlic powder, salt and pepper. Mix well.

3. Spread the chicken and rice mixture evenly into the prepared baking dish. Cover tightly with foil.

4. Bake for 45 minutes. Remove foil and stir in the frozen peas.

5. Sprinkle the shredded cheddar cheese over the top.

6. Return the casserole to the oven and bake for 15 minutes more, until the rice is tender and the cheese is melted and bubbly.

7. Let the casserole stand for 5 minutes before serving.

This chicken and rice casserole is a comforting and easy one•dish meal. The creamy sauce, tender chicken, and cheesy topping make it so satisfying.

You can customize it by using different types of canned soup, adding more vegetables, or topping it with crushed crackers or breadcrumbs. Enjoy!

51. Beef and mushroom stroganoff

Ingredient:

- 1 tsp Dijon mustard
- 1 tsp Worcestershire sauce
- 1 tsp paprika
- Salt and pepper to taste
- 1 cup sour cream
- Chopped parsley for garnish
- Cooked egg noodles, for serving

- 1 lb beef sirloin or tenderloin, cut into 1·inch cubes
- 2 tbsp olive oil
- 1 onion, diced
- 8 oz cremini or button mushrooms, sliced
- 3 cloves garlic, minced
- 2 tbsp tomato paste
- 1 cup beef broth
- 1/2 cup dry white wine

Instructions:

1. In a large skillet or Dutch oven, heat the olive oil over medium·high heat. Working in batches if needed, brown the beef cubes on all sides, about 2·3 minutes per batch. Remove beef to a plate.

2. Reduce heat to medium and add the diced onion to the skillet. Cook for 5·7 minutes until softened.

3. Add the sliced mushrooms and cook for 3·4 minutes until browned.

4. Stir in the minced garlic and tomato paste. Cook for 1 minute.

5. Pour in the beef broth and white wine. Use a wooden spoon to scrape up any browned bits from the bottom of the skillet.

6. Add the Dijon mustard, Worcestershire sauce and paprika. Season with salt and pepper.

7. Return the browned beef and any juices to the skillet. Bring the stroganoff to a simmer, then reduce heat to medium·low. Cover and cook for 20·25 minutes, until the beef is very tender.

8. Remove from heat and stir in the sour cream until well combined.

9. Serve the beef and mushroom stroganoff immediately over cooked egg noodles, garnished with chopped parsley.

The tender beef, earthy mushrooms, and creamy sauce make this stroganoff so rich and satisfying. Adjust the seasoning to your taste.

52. Chicken and broccoli Alfredo

Ingredient:

• 8 oz fettuccine pasta
• 2 boneless, skinless chicken breasts, cubed
• 2 tbsp olive oil
• 1 head of broccoli, cut into florets
• 2 cloves garlic, minced
• 1 cup heavy cream
• 1 cup grated Parmesan cheese
• 2 tbsp butter
• Salt and pepper to taste
• Chopped parsley for garnish

Instructions:

1. Bring a large pot of salted water to a boil. Cook the fettuccine according to package instructions until al dente. Drain and set aside.

2. In a large skillet, heat the olive oil over medium•high heat. Add the cubed chicken and cook for 5•7 minutes, until browned on all sides and cooked through. Remove chicken from the pan and set aside.

3. In the same skillet, add the broccoli florets and a splash of water. Cover and steam the broccoli for 3•5 minutes until tender•crisp. Remove broccoli from the pan.

4. Reduce heat to medium and add the minced garlic to the skillet. Cook for 1 minute until fragrant.

5. Pour in the heavy cream and whisk in the Parmesan cheese. Bring the sauce to a simmer and cook for 2•3 minutes, stirring frequently, until thickened slightly.

6. Reduce heat to low and stir in the butter until melted and incorporated into the sauce.

7. Add the cooked fettuccine, chicken, and broccoli to the sauce. Toss everything together until well coated.

8. Season with salt and pepper to taste.

9. Serve the Chicken and Broccoli Alfredo immediately, garnished with chopped parsley if desired.

53. Beef and potato stew

Ingredient:

- 2 lbs beef stew meat, cut into 1·inch cubes
- 3 tablespoons olive oil
- 1 large onion, diced
- 3 cloves garlic, minced
- 2 tablespoons tomato paste
- 1 cup red wine or beef broth
- 4 cups beef broth
- 2 bay leaves
- 1 teaspoon dried thyme
- Salt and pepper to taste
- 3 medium potatoes, peeled and cut into 1·inch cubes
- 2 carrots, peeled and sliced
- 1 cup frozen peas
- Chopped parsley for garnish

Instructions:

1. In a large pot or Dutch oven, heat the olive oil over medium·high heat. Add the beef cubes and brown on all sides, about 5 minutes total. Remove beef to a plate.

2. Add the onion to the pot and cook for 5 minutes until softened. Add the garlic and tomato paste and cook for 1 minute.

3. Pour in the red wine (or beef broth) and use a wooden spoon to scrape up any browned bits from the bottom of the pot.

4. Add the beef back to the pot along with the beef broth, bay leaves, thyme, salt and pepper. Bring to a boil.

5. Reduce heat to low, cover and simmer for 1 hour, stirring occasionally.

6. Add the potatoes and carrots to the pot. Cover and continue simmering for 30·40 minutes until the vegetables are tender.

7. Stir in the frozen peas and cook for 5 more minutes.

8. Taste and adjust seasoning as needed. Garnish with chopped parsley before serving.

54. Chicken and spinach lasagna

Ingredient:

- 1/2 cup grated Parmesan cheese
- 1 tsp dried basil
- 1/2 tsp dried oregano
- Salt and pepper to taste
- 2 cups shredded mozzarella cheese
- 1 (24 oz) jar marinara sauce
- 2 tbsp olive oil
- 9 lasagna noodles
- 1 lb boneless, skinless chicken breasts, cubed
- 1 onion, diced
- 3 cloves garlic, minced
- 10 oz frozen chopped spinach, thawed and drained
- 15 oz ricotta cheese
- 1 egg

Instructions:

1. Preheat oven to 375°F. Grease a 9x13 inch baking dish.

2. Bring a large pot of salted water to a boil. Cook the lasagna noodles according to package instructions until al dente. Drain and set aside.

3. In a large skillet, heat the olive oil over medium•high heat. Add the cubed chicken and cook for 5•7 minutes, until browned on all sides and cooked through. Remove chicken from the pan and set aside.

4. In the same skillet, add the diced onion and cook for 3•4 minutes until softened. Add the minced garlic and cook for 1 minute until fragrant.

5. Stir the thawed and drained spinach into the onion and garlic mixture. Cook for 2•3 minutes to heat through.

6. In a medium bowl, mix together the ricotta cheese, egg, Parmesan cheese, dried basil, dried oregano, salt and pepper.

7. Spread 1/2 cup of the marinara sauce in the bottom of the prepared baking dish. Layer 3 lasagna noodles in the dish. Spread half of the ricotta cheese mixture over the noodles, then top with half of the chicken and spinach mixture. Sprinkle with 1/2 cup mozzarella cheese.

8. Repeat the layers of noodles, ricotta, chicken/spinach, and mozzarella. Top with the remaining 3 lasagna noodles and the remaining marinara sauce.

9. Cover the dish with aluminum foil and bake for 30 minutes. Remove foil and bake for an additional 15 minutes, until hot and bubbly. Let the lasagna stand for 10 minutes before serving.

55. Beef and vegetable stir·fry

Ingredient:

- 1 lb beef sirloin or flank steak, thinly sliced
- 2 tbsp soy sauce
- 2 tbsp rice vinegar
- 1 tbsp brown sugar
- 2 tsp sesame oil
- 2 tbsp vegetable oil
- 3 cloves garlic, minced
- 1 tbsp grated fresh ginger
- 1 red bell pepper, sliced
- 1 cup broccoli florets
- 1 cup snow peas or snap peas
- 1 cup sliced mushrooms
- 2 green onions, sliced
- Cooked rice, for serving

For the Sauce:

- 2 tbsp soy sauce
- 2 tbsp rice vinegar
- 1 tbsp brown sugar
- 1 tsp cornstarch
- 1/4 cup beef or chicken broth

Instructions:

1. In a medium bowl, combine the sliced beef, 2 tbsp soy sauce, 2 tbsp rice vinegar, 1 tbsp brown sugar, and 2 tsp sesame oil. Toss to coat the beef and let marinate for 15·30 minutes.

2. In a small bowl, whisk together the ingredients for the sauce • 2 tbsp soy sauce, 2 tbsp rice vinegar, 1 tbsp brown sugar, 1 tsp cornstarch, and 1/4 cup broth. Set aside.

3. Heat 1 tbsp vegetable oil in a large skillet or wok over high heat. Add the marinated beef and stir·fry for 2·3 minutes until browned. Remove beef from the pan and set aside.

4. Add the remaining 1 tbsp vegetable oil to the pan. Add the minced garlic and grated ginger and cook for 1 minute until fragrant.

5. Add the sliced bell pepper, broccoli florets, snow peas, and mushrooms to the pan. Stir·fry for 3·4 minutes until the vegetables are crisp·tender.

6. Pour the prepared sauce into the pan and bring to a simmer. Cook for 1·2 minutes until the sauce has thickened slightly.

7. Return the cooked beef to the pan and toss everything together until well combined and heated through.

8. Remove from heat and stir in the sliced green onions.

9. Serve the Beef and Vegetable Stir·Fry immediately over steamed rice.

56. Chicken and mushroom risotto

Ingredient:

- 1 1/2 cups Arborio rice
- 1/2 cup dry white wine
- 1/2 cup grated Parmesan cheese
- 2 tbsp butter
- 2 tbsp chopped fresh parsley
- Salt and pepper to taste

- 4 cups chicken broth
- 2 tbsp olive oil
- 1 lb boneless, skinless chicken thighs, cubed
- 8 oz cremini or button mushrooms, sliced
- 1 onion, diced
- 3 cloves garlic, minced

Instructions:

1. In a saucepan, bring the chicken broth to a simmer and keep it warm over low heat.

2. In a large skillet, heat the olive oil over medium•high heat. Add the cubed chicken and cook for 5•7 minutes, until browned on all sides. Remove the chicken from the pan and set aside.

3. In the same skillet, add the sliced mushrooms and cook for 3•4 minutes until they start to brown. Remove the mushrooms from the pan and set aside with the chicken.

4. Reduce the heat to medium and add the diced onion to the skillet. Cook for 5 minutes, stirring occasionally, until the onion is softened.

5. Add the minced garlic and cook for 1 minute until fragrant.

6. Stir in the Arborio rice and cook for 2•3 minutes, stirring constantly, until the rice is lightly toasted.

7. Pour in the white wine and cook, stirring constantly, until the wine is absorbed, about 2 minutes.

8. Ladle in 1/2 cup of the warm chicken broth and cook, stirring frequently, until the broth is absorbed. Continue this process, adding 1/2 cup of broth at a time, until the rice is tender and creamy, about 20•25 minutes total.

9. Stir the cooked chicken and mushrooms back into the risotto. Cook for 2•3 minutes to heat through.

10. Remove from heat and stir in the Parmesan cheese and butter until melted and incorporated. Season with salt and pepper to taste. Garnish with chopped fresh parsley before serving.

57. Beef and black bean chili

Ingredient:

• 1 lb ground beef
• 1 onion, diced
• 3 cloves garlic, minced
• 2 tbsp chili powder
• 1 tbsp ground cumin
• 1 tsp dried oregano
• 1 tsp smoked paprika
• 1/4 tsp cayenne pepper (or to taste)
• 1 (15 oz) can black beans, drained and rinsed
• 1 (15 oz) can diced tomatoes
• 1 (6 oz) can tomato paste
• 1 cup beef broth
• Salt and pepper to taste
• Shredded cheddar cheese, sour cream, chopped cilantro for serving

Instructions:

1. In a large pot or Dutch oven, cook the ground beef over medium•high heat, breaking it up with a wooden spoon, until browned and cooked through, about 5•7 minutes. Drain any excess fat.

2. Add the diced onion to the pot and cook for 3•4 minutes until softened. Add the minced garlic and cook for 1 minute until fragrant.

3. Stir in the chili powder, cumin, oregano, smoked paprika, and cayenne pepper. Cook for 1•2 minutes to toast the spices.

4. Pour in the drained and rinsed black beans, diced tomatoes, tomato paste, and beef broth. Stir to combine.

5. Bring the chili to a simmer and let it cook for 20•25 minutes, stirring occasionally, until thickened to your desired consistency.

6. Taste and season with salt and pepper as needed. Serve the Beef and Black Bean Chili hot, topped with shredded cheddar cheese, a dollop of sour cream, and chopped fresh cilantro.

This hearty chili is packed with bold flavors from the spices and the tender beef and black beans. It's perfect for a cozy meal on a chilly day. Enjoy!

58. Chicken and corn chowder

Ingredient:

• 2 boneless, skinless chicken breasts, cubed
• 2 tbsp olive oil
• 1 onion, diced
• 2 celery stalks, diced
• 2 carrots, peeled and diced
• 3 cloves garlic, minced
• 4 cups chicken broth
• 2 medium potatoes, peeled and diced
• 2 cups frozen corn kernels
• 1 cup heavy cream
• 2 tbsp butter
• 1 tsp dried thyme
• Salt and pepper to taste
• Chopped parsley for garnish

Instructions:

1. In a large pot or Dutch oven, heat the olive oil over medium•high heat. Add the cubed chicken and cook for 5•7 minutes, until browned on all sides and cooked through. Remove chicken from the pot and set aside.

2. In the same pot, add the diced onion, celery, and carrots. Cook for 5•7 minutes, stirring occasionally, until the vegetables are softened.

3. Add the minced garlic and cook for 1 minute until fragrant.

4. Pour in the chicken broth and add the diced potatoes. Bring the mixture to a boil, then reduce heat and simmer for 10•15 minutes, until the potatoes are tender.

5. Stir in the frozen corn kernels and the cooked chicken. Simmer for 5 more minutes.

6. Reduce heat to low and stir in the heavy cream and butter. Cook for 2•3 minutes, stirring frequently, until the butter is melted and the chowder has thickened slightly.

7. Season with the dried thyme, salt, and pepper to taste. Ladle the Chicken and Corn Chowder into bowls and garnish with chopped parsley before serving.

59. Beef and barley soup

Ingredient:

- 1 lb beef stew meat, cut into 1•inch cubes
- 2 tbsp olive oil
- 1 onion, diced
- 3 carrots, peeled and sliced
- 3 celery stalks, sliced
- 4 cloves garlic, minced
- 8 cups beef broth
- 1 cup pearl barley
- 1 (14.5 oz) can diced tomatoes
- 2 bay leaves
- 1 tsp dried thyme
- Salt and pepper to taste
- Chopped parsley for garnish

Instructions:

1. In a large pot or Dutch oven, heat the olive oil over medium•high heat. Add the beef cubes and brown on all sides, about 5 minutes total. Remove beef to a plate.

2. Add the diced onion, sliced carrots, and sliced celery to the pot. Cook for 5•7 minutes, stirring occasionally, until the vegetables start to soften.

3. Add the minced garlic and cook for 1 minute until fragrant.

4. Pour in the beef broth and add the pearl barley, diced tomatoes, bay leaves, and dried thyme. Stir to combine.

5. Return the browned beef cubes to the pot. Bring the soup to a boil, then reduce heat and let it simmer for 45•60 minutes, until the barley is tender and the beef is very tender.

6. Remove the bay leaves. Season the soup with salt and pepper to taste.

7. Ladle the Beef and Barley Soup into bowls and garnish with chopped parsley before serving.

This hearty and comforting soup is perfect for a chilly day. The barley adds great texture and the beef makes it nice and filling. Enjoy!

60. Chicken and sweet potato curry

Ingredient:

• 1 lb boneless, skinless chicken thighs, cubed
• 2 tbsp olive oil
• 1 onion, diced
• 3 cloves garlic, minced
• 1 tbsp grated fresh ginger
• 2 tsp garam masala
• 1 tsp ground cumin
• 1 tsp ground coriander
• 1 tsp turmeric
• 1/4 tsp cayenne pepper (or to taste)
• 1 (14 oz) can diced tomatoes
• 1 (13.5 oz) can coconut milk
• 2 medium sweet potatoes, peeled and cubed
• 1 cup frozen peas
• Salt and pepper to taste
• Chopped cilantro for garnish

Instructions:

1. In a large skillet or Dutch oven, heat the olive oil over medium•high heat. Add the cubed chicken and cook for 5•7 minutes, until browned on all sides. Remove chicken from the pan and set aside.

2. In the same pan, add the diced onion and cook for 3•4 minutes until softened. Add the minced garlic and grated ginger and cook for 1 minute until fragrant.

3. Stir in the garam masala, cumin, coriander, turmeric, and cayenne pepper. Cook for 1 minute to toast the spices.

4. Pour in the diced tomatoes and coconut milk. Bring the mixture to a simmer.

5. Add the cubed sweet potatoes to the pan and return the cooked chicken to the curry. Reduce heat to medium•low, cover and simmer for 15•20 minutes, until the sweet potatoes are tender.

6. Stir in the frozen peas and cook for 5 more minutes. Season the curry with salt and pepper to taste. Serve the Chicken and Sweet Potato Curry over basmati rice, garnished with chopped cilantro.

61. Beef and vegetable curry

Ingredient:

- 1 lb beef stew meat, cut into 1•inch cubes
- 2 tbsp vegetable oil
- 1 onion, diced
- 3 cloves garlic, minced
- 1 tbsp grated fresh ginger
- 2 tsp garam masala
- 1 tsp ground cumin
- 1 tsp ground coriander
- 1 tsp turmeric
- 1/2 tsp cayenne pepper (or to taste)
- 1 (14 oz) can diced tomatoes
- 1 (13.5 oz) can coconut milk
- 2 medium potatoes, peeled and cubed
- 1 cup cauliflower florets
- 1 cup frozen peas
- Salt and pepper to taste
- Chopped cilantro for garnish

Instructions:

1. In a large skillet or Dutch oven, heat the vegetable oil over medium•high heat. Add the beef cubes and cook for 5•7 minutes, until browned on all sides. Remove beef from the pan and set aside.

2. In the same pan, add the diced onion and cook for 3•4 minutes until softened. Add the minced garlic and grated ginger and cook for 1 minute until fragrant.

3. Stir in the garam masala, cumin, coriander, turmeric, and cayenne pepper. Cook for 1 minute to toast the spices.

4. Pour in the diced tomatoes and coconut milk. Bring the mixture to a simmer.

5. Add the cubed potatoes and cauliflower florets to the pan and return the cooked beef to the curry. Reduce heat to medium•low, cover and simmer for 20•25 minutes, until the vegetables are tender.

6. Stir in the frozen peas and cook for 5 more minutes.

7. Season the curry with salt and pepper to taste.

8. Serve the Beef and Vegetable Curry over basmati rice, garnished with chopped cilantro.

This flavorful curry is packed with tender beef and an assortment of vegetables in a rich, creamy coconut milk sauce. It's a delicious and comforting meal. Enjoy!

62. Chicken and vegetable kebabs

Ingredient:

• 1 lb boneless, skinless chicken breasts, cut into 1•inch cubes
• 1 red bell pepper, cut into 1•inch pieces
• 1 yellow bell pepper, cut into 1•inch pieces
• 1 red onion, cut into 1•inch pieces
• 8 oz mushrooms, halved
• 1 zucchini, cut into 1•inch pieces
• Wooden or metal skewers

Marinade:
• 1/4 cup olive oil
• 2 tbsp lemon juice
• 2 cloves garlic, minced
• 1 tsp dried oregano
• 1 tsp dried basil
• Salt and pepper to taste

Instructions:

1. In a large bowl, whisk together the ingredients for the marinade • olive oil, lemon juice, garlic, oregano, basil, salt and pepper.

2. Add the cubed chicken, bell pepper pieces, onion, mushrooms, and zucchini to the marinade and toss to coat everything evenly. Cover and refrigerate for 30 minutes to 1 hour.

3. Preheat grill or grill pan to medium•high heat.

4. Thread the marinated chicken and vegetables onto the skewers, alternating the ingredients.

5. Grill the kebabs for 12•15 minutes total, turning occasionally, until the chicken is cooked through and the vegetables are tender.

6. Serve the Chicken and Vegetable Kebabs immediately, with any extra marinade drizzled over the top.

Tips:
• Soak wooden skewers in water for 30 minutes before using to prevent burning.
• Cut the vegetables into similar•sized pieces so they cook evenly.

63. Beef and cheese enchiladas

Ingredient:

- 1 lb ground beef
- 1 onion, diced
- 3 cloves garlic, minced
- 1 tbsp chili powder
- 1 tsp cumin
- 1 tsp oregano
- Salt and pepper to taste
- 12 corn tortillas
- 2 cups shredded cheddar cheese
- 1 (15 oz) can enchilada sauce

For the Enchilada Sauce:

- 2 tbsp olive oil
- 2 tbsp all•purpose flour
- 2 cups chicken or beef broth
- 1 (8 oz) can tomato sauce
- 1 tsp chili powder
- 1 tsp cumin
- 1/2 tsp garlic powder
- Salt and pepper to taste

Instructions:

1. Preheat oven to 375°F. Grease a 9x13 inch baking dish.

2. In a large skillet, cook the ground beef over medium•high heat until browned and crumbled. Drain excess fat.

3. Add the diced onion and minced garlic to the skillet. Cook for 3•4 minutes until onions are translucent.

4. Stir in the chili powder, cumin, oregano, salt and pepper. Cook for 1 minute.

5. To make the enchilada sauce, heat the olive oil in a saucepan over medium heat. Whisk in the flour and cook for 1 minute.

6. Gradually whisk in the broth, tomato sauce, chili powder, cumin, garlic powder, salt and pepper. Bring to a simmer and cook for 5•7 minutes until thickened.

7. Spread 1/2 cup of the enchilada sauce in the bottom of the prepared baking dish.

8. Warm the corn tortillas according to package instructions. Spoon about 2•3 tbsp of the beef mixture onto each tortilla. Roll up tightly and place seam•side down in the baking dish.

9. Pour the remaining enchilada sauce over the rolled enchiladas. Top with the shredded cheddar cheese. Bake for 20•25 minutes until hot and bubbly.Serve the beef and cheese enchiladas warm, garnished with chopped cilantro if desired

64. Chicken and avocado wraps

Ingredient:

• 2 boneless, skinless chicken breasts
• 1 tbsp olive oil
• 1 tsp chili powder
• 1/2 tsp cumin
• Salt and pepper to taste
• 2 avocados, pitted and sliced
• 1 cup shredded romaine lettuce
• 1/2 cup diced tomatoes
• 1/4 cup crumbled feta cheese
• 4•6 large tortilla or wrap shells

Dressing:

• 2 tbsp olive oil
• 1 tbsp lime juice
• 1 tbsp chopped cilantro
• 1 tsp honey
• Salt and pepper to taste

Instructions:

1. Preheat oven to 400°F. Line a baking sheet with foil.

2. Place the chicken breasts on the prepared baking sheet. Drizzle with 1 tbsp olive oil and sprinkle with chili powder, cumin, salt and pepper.

3. Bake the chicken for 20•25 minutes, until cooked through. Allow to cool slightly, then shred or dice the chicken.

4. In a small bowl, whisk together the ingredients for the dressing • olive oil, lime juice, cilantro, honey, salt and pepper.

5. To assemble the wraps, place a tortilla or wrap shell on a flat surface. Layer with some of the shredded chicken, sliced avocado, shredded romaine, diced tomatoes, and crumbled feta cheese.

6. Drizzle the dressing over the fillings.

7. Fold the bottom of the wrap up over the fillings, then fold in the sides and continue rolling up tightly to form a wrap.

8. Repeat with the remaining ingredients to make 4•6 wraps. Serve the Chicken and Avocado Wraps immediately.

These wraps are packed with flavorful grilled chicken, creamy avocado, fresh veggies, and a tangy lime•cilantro dressing. They make a delicious and healthy lunch or light dinner. Enjoy!

65. Beef and vegetable stir·fry

Ingredient:

- 1 lb beef sirloin or flank steak, thinly sliced
- 2 tbsp soy sauce, divided
- 2 tsp cornstarch, divided
- 2 tbsp vegetable oil, divided
- 1 red bell pepper, sliced
- 1 cup broccoli florets
- 1 cup snow peas or snap peas
- 8 oz mushrooms, sliced
- 3 cloves garlic, minced
- 1 tbsp grated fresh ginger
- 1/4 cup beef or chicken broth
- 2 tbsp brown sugar
- 1 tbsp rice vinegar
- 1 tsp sesame oil
- Salt and pepper to taste
- Cooked rice, for serving

Instructions:

1. In a medium bowl, combine the sliced beef, 1 tbsp soy sauce, and 1 tsp cornstarch. Toss to coat the beef and let marinate for 15·30 minutes.

2. In a small bowl, whisk together the remaining 1 tbsp soy sauce, 1 tsp cornstarch, broth, brown sugar, rice vinegar, and sesame oil. Set aside.

3. Heat 1 tbsp vegetable oil in a large skillet or wok over high heat. Add the marinated beef and stir·fry for 2·3 minutes until browned. Remove beef from the pan and set aside.

4. Add the remaining 1 tbsp vegetable oil to the pan. Add the sliced bell pepper, broccoli florets, snow peas, and mushrooms. Stir·fry for 3·4 minutes until the vegetables are crisp·tender.

5. Push the vegetables to the sides of the pan and add the minced garlic and grated ginger to the center. Cook for 1 minute until fragrant.

6. Pour the sauce mixture into the pan and bring to a simmer. Cook for 1·2 minutes until the sauce has thickened slightly.

7. Return the cooked beef to the pan and toss everything together until well combined and heated through.

8. Season with salt and pepper to taste.

9. Serve the Beef and Vegetable Stir·Fry immediately over steamed rice.

This quick and flavorful stir·fry is packed with tender beef and a variety of crisp vegetables, all coated in a savory, slightly sweet sauce. Enjoy!

66. Chicken and black bean burritos

Ingredient:

• 1 lb boneless,
skinless chicken breasts, cubed
• 1 tbsp olive oil
• 1 onion, diced
• 3 cloves garlic, minced
• 1 tbsp chili powder
• 1 tsp ground cumin

• 1 (15 oz) can black beans, drained and rinsed
• 1 cup cooked rice
• 1 cup shredded cheddar or Monterey Jack cheese
• 8•10 large flour tortillas
• Toppings: salsa, sour cream, shredded lettuce, diced tomatoes, etc.

Instructions:

1. In a large skillet, heat the olive oil over medium•high heat. Add the cubed chicken and cook for 5•7 minutes, until browned on all sides and cooked through. Remove chicken from the pan and set aside.

2. In the same skillet, add the diced onion and cook for 3•4 minutes until softened. Add the minced garlic and cook for 1 minute until fragrant.

3. Stir in the chili powder and cumin. Cook for 1 minute to toast the spices.

4. Add the drained and rinsed black beans and the cooked chicken back to the skillet. Stir to combine and cook for 2•3 minutes to heat through.

5. Remove the skillet from heat and stir in the cooked rice and 1/2 cup of the shredded cheese.

6. Warm the flour tortillas according to package instructions.

7. Spoon the chicken and black bean mixture down the center of each tortilla. Top with additional shredded cheese, if desired.

8. Fold the bottom of the tortilla up over the filling, then fold in the sides and continue rolling up tightly to form a burrito.

9. Serve the Chicken and Black Bean Burritos warm, with desired toppings such as salsa, sour cream, shredded lettuce, and diced tomatoes.

These hearty burritos are packed with seasoned chicken, black beans, rice, and melty cheese. They make a satisfying and delicious meal! Enjoy.

67. Beef and broccoli stir·fry

Ingredient:

- 3 cloves garlic, minced
- 1 tbsp grated fresh ginger
- 1/4 cup beef broth
- 2 tbsp brown sugar
- 1 tbsp rice vinegar
- 1 tsp sesame oil
- Salt and pepper to taste
- Cooked rice, for serving

- 1 lb flank steak or sirloin, thinly sliced against the grain
- 2 tbsp soy sauce, divided
- 2 tsp cornstarch, divided
- 2 tbsp vegetable oil, divided
- 3 cups broccoli florets

Instructions:

1. In a medium bowl, combine the sliced beef, 1 tbsp soy sauce, and 1 tsp cornstarch. Toss to coat the beef and let marinate for 15·30 minutes.

2. In a small bowl, whisk together the remaining 1 tbsp soy sauce, 1 tsp cornstarch, beef broth, brown sugar, rice vinegar, and sesame oil. Set aside.

3. Heat 1 tbsp vegetable oil in a large skillet or wok over high heat. Add the marinated beef and stir·fry for 2·3 minutes until browned. Remove beef from the pan and set aside.

4. Add the remaining 1 tbsp vegetable oil to the pan. Add the broccoli florets and stir·fry for 3·4 minutes until crisp·tender.

5. Push the broccoli to the sides of the pan and add the minced garlic and grated ginger to the center. Cook for 1 minute until fragrant.

6. Pour the sauce mixture into the pan and bring to a simmer. Cook for 1·2 minutes until the sauce has thickened slightly.

7. Return the cooked beef to the pan and toss everything together until well combined and heated through.

8. Season with salt and pepper to taste. Serve the Beef and Broccoli Stir·Fry immediately over steamed rice.

This quick and flavorful stir·fry is a great weeknight meal. The tender beef and crisp broccoli are coated in a savory, slightly sweet sauce. Enjoy!

68. Chicken and pineapple fried rice

Ingredient:

• 2 boneless, skinless chicken breasts, cubed
• 2 tbsp vegetable oil, divided
• 2 eggs, beaten
• 1 onion, diced
• 3 cloves garlic, minced
• 1 cup frozen peas and carrots
• 3 cups cooked and chilled rice
• 1 cup diced pineapple
• 2 tbsp soy sauce
• 1 tsp sesame oil
• Salt and pepper to taste
• Chopped green onions for garnish

Instructions:

1. In a large skillet or wok, heat 1 tbsp of the vegetable oil over medium•high heat. Add the cubed chicken and cook for 5•7 minutes, until browned on all sides and cooked through. Remove the chicken from the pan and set aside.

2. In the same pan, add the remaining 1 tbsp of vegetable oil. Pour in the beaten eggs and scramble them, breaking them up into small pieces as they cook. Remove the eggs from the pan and set aside.

3. Add the diced onion to the pan and cook for 3•4 minutes until softened. Add the minced garlic and cook for 1 minute until fragrant.

4. Stir in the frozen peas and carrots and cook for 2•3 minutes until heated through.

5. Add the cooked and chilled rice to the pan. Use a spatula to break up any clumps and stir the rice to coat it in the vegetable mixture.

6. Add the cooked chicken, scrambled eggs, diced pineapple, soy sauce, and sesame oil. Toss everything together until well combined and heated through.

7. Season the fried rice with salt and pepper to taste. Serve the Chicken and Pineapple Fried Rice hot, garnished with chopped green onions.

The sweet pineapple pairs so nicely with the savory chicken and vegetables in this flavorful fried rice dish. It's a great way to use up leftover rice! Enjoy.

69. Beef and potato curry

Ingredient:

• 1 lb beef stew meat, cut into 1•inch cubes
• 2 tbsp vegetable oil
• 1 onion, diced
• 3 cloves garlic, minced
• 1 tbsp grated fresh ginger
• 2 tsp garam masala
• 1 tsp ground cumin
• 1 tsp ground coriander
• 1 tsp turmeric
• 1/2 tsp cayenne pepper (or to taste)
• 1 (14 oz) can diced tomatoes
• 1 (13.5 oz) can coconut milk
• 2 medium potatoes, peeled and cubed
• Salt and pepper to taste
• Chopped cilantro for garnish
• Cooked basmati rice, for serving

Instructions:

1. In a large skillet or Dutch oven, heat the vegetable oil over medium•high heat. Add the beef cubes and cook for 5•7 minutes, until browned on all sides. Remove beef from the pan and set aside.

2. In the same pan, add the diced onion and cook for 3•4 minutes until softened. Add the minced garlic and grated ginger and cook for 1 minute until fragrant.

3. Stir in the garam masala, cumin, coriander, turmeric, and cayenne pepper. Cook for 1 minute to toast the spices.

4. Pour in the diced tomatoes and coconut milk. Bring the mixture to a simmer.

5. Add the cubed potatoes to the pan and return the cooked beef to the curry. Reduce heat to medium•low, cover and simmer for 20•25 minutes, until the potatoes are tender.

6. Season the curry with salt and pepper to taste. Serve the Beef and Potato Curry over basmati rice, garnished with chopped cilantro.

The tender beef and potatoes are simmered in a rich, aromatic coconut milk•based curry sauce. It's a comforting and flavorful dish that pairs perfectly with the fluffy basmati rice.

70. Chicken and vegetable curry

Ingredient:

- 1 tsp ground coriander
- 1 tsp turmeric
- 1/2 tsp cayenne pepper (or to taste)
- 1 (14 oz) can diced tomatoes
- 1 (13.5 oz) can coconut milk
- 2 medium potatoes, peeled and cubed
- 1 cup cauliflower florets
- 1 cup frozen peas
- Salt and pepper to taste
- Chopped cilantro for garnish
- 1 lb boneless, skinless chicken thighs, cut into 1•inch pieces
- 2 tbsp vegetable oil
- 1 onion, diced
- 3 cloves garlic, minced
- 1 tbsp grated fresh ginger
- 2 tsp garam masala
- 1 tsp ground cumin

Instructions:

1. In a large skillet or Dutch oven, heat the vegetable oil over medium•high heat. Add the cubed chicken and cook for 5•7 minutes, until browned on all sides. Remove chicken from the pan and set aside.

2. In the same pan, add the diced onion and cook for 3•4 minutes until softened. Add the minced garlic and grated ginger and cook for 1 minute until fragrant.

3. Stir in the garam masala, cumin, coriander, turmeric, and cayenne pepper. Cook for 1 minute to toast the spices.

4. Pour in the diced tomatoes and coconut milk. Bring the mixture to a simmer.

5. Add the cubed potatoes and cauliflower florets to the pan and return the cooked chicken to the curry. Reduce heat to medium•low, cover and simmer for 20•25 minutes, until the vegetables are tender.

6. Stir in the frozen peas and cook for 5 more minutes.

7. Season the curry with salt and pepper to taste.

8. Serve the Chicken and Vegetable Curry over basmati rice, garnished with chopped cilantro.

This flavorful curry is packed with tender chicken, potatoes, cauliflower, and peas in a rich, creamy coconut milk sauce. It's a delicious and comforting meal. Enjoy

71. Beef and cheese quesadillas

Ingredient:

- 1 lb ground beef
- 1 onion, diced
- 2 cloves garlic, minced
- 1 tbsp chili powder
- 1 tsp ground cumin
- 1/2 tsp dried oregano
- Salt and pepper to taste
- 8 large flour tortillas
- 2 cups shredded cheddar or Monterey Jack cheese
- Butter or oil for cooking

Toppings (optional):
- Salsa
- Sour cream
- Guacamole
- Diced tomatoes
- Shredded lettuce

Instructions:

1. In a large skillet, cook the ground beef over medium·high heat, breaking it up with a wooden spoon, until browned and cooked through, about 5·7 minutes. Drain any excess fat.

2. Add the diced onion to the skillet and cook for 3·4 minutes until softened. Add the minced garlic and cook for 1 minute until fragrant.

3. Stir in the chili powder, cumin, oregano, and a pinch of salt and pepper. Cook for 1·2 minutes to toast the spices.

4. Remove the beef mixture from the heat and set aside.

5. Heat a large skillet or griddle over medium heat. Lightly butter or oil the surface.

6. Place one tortilla in the pan and top with 1/4 of the beef mixture and 1/4 cup of the shredded cheese. Top with another tortilla.

7. Cook the quesadilla for 2·3 minutes per side, until the tortilla is lightly browned and the cheese is melted.

8. Repeat with the remaining tortillas, beef, and cheese to make 4 quesadillas total.

9. Cut each quesadilla into wedges and serve warm, with desired toppings like salsa, sour cream, guacamole, diced tomatoes, and shredded lettuce.

These Beef and Cheese Quesadillas are a quick and easy meal that's packed with flavor. The seasoned ground beef and melty cheese make them irresistible. Enjoy!

72. Chicken and vegetable stir·fry

Ingredient:

- 3 cloves garlic, minced
- 1 tbsp grated fresh ginger
- 1/4 cup chicken broth
- 2 tbsp brown sugar
- 1 tbsp rice vinegar
- 1 tsp sesame oil
- Salt and pepper to taste
- Cooked rice, for serving

- 1 lb boneless, skinless chicken breasts, cut into 1·inch pieces
- 2 tbsp soy sauce, divided
- 2 tsp cornstarch, divided
- 2 tbsp vegetable oil, divided
- 1 red bell pepper, sliced
- 1 cup broccoli florets
- 1 cup snow peas or snap peas
- 8 oz mushrooms, sliced

Instructions:

1. In a medium bowl, combine the cubed chicken, 1 tbsp soy sauce, and 1 tsp cornstarch. Toss to coat the chicken and let marinate for 15·30 minutes.

2. In a small bowl, whisk together the remaining 1 tbsp soy sauce, 1 tsp cornstarch, chicken broth, brown sugar, rice vinegar, and sesame oil. Set aside.

3. Heat 1 tbsp vegetable oil in a large skillet or wok over high heat. Add the marinated chicken and stir·fry for 3·4 minutes until browned. Remove chicken from the pan and set aside.

4. Add the remaining 1 tbsp vegetable oil to the pan. Add the sliced bell pepper, broccoli florets, snow peas, and mushrooms. Stir·fry for 4·5 minutes until the vegetables are crisp·tender.

5. Push the vegetables to the sides of the pan and add the minced garlic and grated ginger to the center. Cook for 1 minute until fragrant.

6. Pour the sauce mixture into the pan and bring to a simmer. Cook for 1·2 minutes until the sauce has thickened slightly.

7. Return the cooked chicken to the pan and toss everything together until well combined and heated through.

8. Season with salt and pepper to taste. Serve the Chicken and Vegetable Stir·Fry immediately over steamed rice.

This quick and flavorful stir·fry is packed with tender chicken and a variety of crisp vegetables, all coated in a savory, slightly sweet sauce. Enjoy!

73. Beef and bean burritos

Ingredient:

- 1 lb ground beef
- 1 onion, diced
- 3 cloves garlic, minced
- 1 tbsp chili powder
- 1 tsp ground cumin
- 1 tsp dried oregano
- 1/2 tsp smoked paprika
- Salt and pepper to taste
- 1 (15 oz) can black beans, drained and rinsed
- 1 cup shredded cheddar cheese
- 8•10 large flour tortillas
- Toppings: salsa, sour cream, shredded lettuce, diced tomatoes, etc.

Instructions:

1. In a large skillet, cook the ground beef over medium•high heat, breaking it up with a wooden spoon, until browned and cooked through, about 5•7 minutes. Drain any excess fat.

2. Add the diced onion to the skillet and cook for 3•4 minutes until softened. Add the minced garlic and cook for 1 minute until fragrant.

3. Stir in the chili powder, cumin, oregano, smoked paprika, and a pinch of salt and pepper. Cook for 1•2 minutes to toast the spices.

4. Add the drained and rinsed black beans to the skillet and stir to combine with the beef mixture. Cook for 2•3 minutes to heat through.

5. Remove the skillet from heat and stir in 1/2 cup of the shredded cheddar cheese.

6. Warm the flour tortillas according to package instructions.

7. Spoon the beef and bean mixture down the center of each tortilla. Top with additional shredded cheese, if desired.

8. Fold the bottom of the tortilla up over the filling, then fold in the sides and continue rolling up tightly to form a burrito.

9. Serve the beef and bean burritos warm, with desired toppings such as salsa, sour cream, shredded lettuce, and diced tomatoes.

These hearty burritos are packed with seasoned ground beef, black beans, and melty cheese. They make a satisfying and delicious meal! Enjoy.

74. Chicken and rice casserole

Ingredient:

• 1 lb boneless, skinless chicken breasts, cut into 1•inch pieces
• 1 cup uncooked long•grain white rice
• 1 (10.5 oz) can cream of mushroom soup
• 1 (10.5 oz) can cream of chicken soup
• 1 cup chicken broth
• 1/2 cup milk
• 1 tsp garlic powder
• 1 tsp onion powder
• 1/2 tsp dried thyme
• Salt and pepper to taste
• 1 cup frozen peas
• 1 cup shredded cheddar cheese

Instructions:

1. Preheat oven to 375°F. Grease a 9x13 inch baking dish.

2. In a large bowl, combine the chicken, uncooked rice, cream of mushroom soup, cream of chicken soup, chicken broth, milk, garlic powder, onion powder, thyme, salt and pepper. Mix well.

3. Spread the chicken and rice mixture evenly into the prepared baking dish. Cover tightly with foil.

4. Bake for 45 minutes. Remove foil, stir in the frozen peas, and sprinkle the shredded cheddar cheese on top.

5. Return to the oven and bake for 15 more minutes, until the rice is tender and the cheese is melted and bubbly.

6. Let stand for 5 minutes before serving.

Serve the chicken and rice casserole warm. Enjoy!

This is a simple, comforting one•dish meal that's perfect for busy weeknights. The creamy sauce, tender chicken, and cheesy topping make it a family favorite.

75. Beef and mushroom stroganoff

Ingredient:

- 1 lb beef sirloin or tenderloin, cut into 1·inch cubes
- 2 tbsp olive oil
- 1 onion, diced
- 8 oz mushrooms, sliced
- 2 cloves garlic, minced
- 1 tbsp tomato paste
- 1 cup beef broth
- 1/2 cup dry white wine or sherry
- 1 tsp Dijon mustard
- 1 tsp Worcestershire sauce
- 1 bay leaf
- 1 tsp paprika
- Salt and pepper to taste
- 1 cup sour cream
- 2 tbsp chopped fresh parsley
- Cooked egg noodles, for serving

Instructions:

1. In a large skillet, heat the olive oil over medium·high heat. Add the beef cubes and brown on all sides, about 5 minutes total. Remove beef to a plate.

2. Add the onions to the skillet and cook for 5 minutes until softened. Add the mushrooms and garlic and cook for 2·3 minutes more.

3. Stir in the tomato paste and cook for 1 minute.

4. Pour in the beef broth and white wine. Add the Dijon, Worcestershire, bay leaf, paprika, salt and pepper. Bring to a simmer.

5. Return the seared beef and any juices to the skillet. Reduce heat to low, cover and simmer for 45·60 minutes, until beef is very tender.

6. Remove the bay leaf. Stir in the sour cream and heat through, but do not boil.

7. Taste and adjust seasoning as needed. Stir in the chopped parsley.

8. Serve the beef stroganoff immediately over cooked egg noodles.

76. Chicken and broccoli Alfredo

Ingredient:

• 8 oz fettuccine pasta
• 1 lb boneless, skinless chicken breasts, cubed
• 2 tbsp olive oil
• 1 head of broccoli, cut into florets
• 2 cloves garlic, minced
• 1 cup heavy cream
• 1 cup grated Parmesan cheese
• 2 tbsp butter
• Salt and pepper to taste
• Chopped parsley for garnish

Instructions:

1. Bring a large pot of salted water to a boil. Cook the fettuccine according to package instructions until al dente. Drain and set aside.

2. In a large skillet, heat the olive oil over medium•high heat. Add the cubed chicken and cook for 5•7 minutes, until browned on all sides and cooked through. Remove chicken from the pan and set aside.

3. In the same skillet, add the broccoli florets and a splash of water. Cover and steam the broccoli for 3•5 minutes until tender•crisp. Remove broccoli from the pan.

4. Reduce heat to medium and add the minced garlic to the skillet. Cook for 1 minute until fragrant.

5. Pour in the heavy cream and whisk in the Parmesan cheese. Bring the sauce to a simmer and cook for 2•3 minutes, stirring frequently, until thickened slightly.

6. Reduce heat to low and stir in the butter until melted and incorporated into the sauce.

7. Add the cooked fettuccine, chicken, and broccoli to the sauce. Toss everything together until well coated.

8. Season with salt and pepper to taste. Serve the Chicken and Broccoli Alfredo immediately, garnished with chopped parsley if desired.

Enjoy this rich and creamy Alfredo dish! The tender chicken and broccoli pair perfectly with the indulgent Parmesan sauce. Let me know if you have any other questions.

77. Beef and potato stew

Ingredient:

• 2 lbs beef stew meat, cut into 1•inch cubes
• 3 tablespoons olive oil
• 1 large onion, diced
• 3 cloves garlic, minced
• 2 tablespoons tomato paste
• 1 cup red wine or beef broth
• 4 cups beef broth
• 2 bay leaves
• 1 teaspoon dried thyme
• Salt and pepper to taste
• 3 medium potatoes, peeled and cut into 1•inch cubes
• 2 carrots, peeled and sliced
• 1 cup frozen peas

Instructions:

1. In a large pot or Dutch oven, heat the olive oil over medium•high heat. Add the beef cubes and brown on all sides, about 5 minutes total. Remove beef to a plate.

2. Add the onion to the pot and cook for 5 minutes until softened. Add the garlic and tomato paste and cook for 1 minute.

3. Pour in the red wine (or beef broth) and use a wooden spoon to scrape up any browned bits from the bottom of the pot.

4. Add the beef back to the pot along with the beef broth, bay leaves, thyme, salt and pepper. Bring to a boil.

5. Reduce heat to low, cover and simmer for 1 hour.

6. Add the potatoes and carrots. Cover and simmer for 30•40 minutes more, until beef and vegetables are very tender.

7. Stir in the frozen peas and cook for 5 more minutes.

8. Taste and adjust seasoning as needed. Serve hot.

78. Chicken and spinach lasagna

Ingredient:

- 9 lasagna noodles
- 2 tbsp olive oil
- 1 tsp dried basil
- 1/2 tsp dried oregano
- Salt and pepper to taste
- 2 cups shredded mozzarella cheese
- 1 (24 oz) jar marinara sauce
- 1 lb boneless, skinless chicken breasts, cubed
- 1 onion, diced
- 3 cloves garlic, minced
- 10 oz frozen chopped spinach, thawed and drained
- 15 oz ricotta cheese
- 1 egg
- 1/2 cup grated Parmesan cheese

Instructions:

1. Preheat oven to 375°F. Grease a 9x13 inch baking dish.

2. Bring a large pot of salted water to a boil. Cook the lasagna noodles according to package instructions until al dente. Drain and set aside.

3. In a large skillet, heat the olive oil over medium•high heat. Add the cubed chicken and cook for 5•7 minutes, until browned on all sides and cooked through. Remove chicken from the pan and set aside.

4. In the same skillet, add the diced onion and cook for 3•4 minutes until softened. Add the minced garlic and cook for 1 minute until fragrant.

5. Stir the thawed and drained spinach into the onion and garlic mixture. Cook for 2•3 minutes to heat through.

6. In a medium bowl, mix together the ricotta cheese, egg, Parmesan cheese, dried basil, dried oregano, salt and pepper.

7. Spread 1/2 cup of the marinara sauce in the bottom of the prepared baking dish.

8. Layer 3 lasagna noodles in the dish. Spread half of the ricotta cheese mixture over the noodles, then top with half of the chicken and spinach mixture. Sprinkle with 1/2 cup mozzarella cheese.

9. Repeat the layers of noodles, ricotta, chicken/spinach, and mozzarella. Top with the remaining 3 lasagna noodles and the remaining marinara sauce. Cover the dish with aluminum foil and bake for 30 minutes. Remove foil and bake for an additional 15 minutes, until hot and bubbly. Let the lasagna stand for 10 minutes before serving.

79. Beef and vegetable stir·fry

Ingredient:

• 1 lb beef sirloin or flank steak, thinly sliced
• 2 tbsp vegetable oil
• 1 red bell pepper, sliced
• 1 cup broccoli florets
• 1 cup sliced mushrooms
• 1 cup snow peas or snap peas
• 3 cloves garlic, minced
• 1 tbsp grated fresh ginger
• 2 tbsp soy sauce
• 1 tbsp rice vinegar
• 1 tsp sesame oil
• 1 tsp cornstarch
• Salt and pepper to taste
• Cooked rice, for serving

Instructions:

1. In a small bowl, whisk together the soy sauce, rice vinegar, sesame oil, and cornstarch. Set aside.

2. Heat the vegetable oil in a large skillet or wok over high heat. Add the beef and stir·fry for 2·3 minutes until browned on the edges but still pink in the center. Remove beef to a plate.

3. Add the bell pepper, broccoli, mushrooms, and snow peas to the hot pan. Stir·fry for 3·4 minutes until vegetables are crisp·tender.

4. Add the garlic and ginger and cook for 1 minute, stirring constantly.

5. Return the beef and any juices to the pan. Pour in the soy sauce mixture and toss everything together until the sauce thickens, about 1·2 minutes.

6. Remove from heat and season with salt and pepper to taste.

7. Serve the beef and vegetable stir·fry immediately over steamed rice.

This quick and easy stir·fry is packed with tender beef, fresh vegetables, and a savory sauce. It's a great weeknight meal that's ready in under 30 minutes!

80. Chicken and mushroom risotto

Ingredient:

• 4 cups chicken broth
• 2 tbsp olive oil
• 1 lb boneless, skinless chicken breasts, cut into 1•inch pieces
• 8 oz cremini or button mushrooms, sliced
• 1 onion, diced
• 2 cloves garlic, minced
• 1 1/2 cups Arborio rice
• 1/2 cup dry white wine
• 1/2 cup grated Parmesan cheese
• 2 tbsp butter
• 2 tbsp chopped fresh parsley
• Salt and pepper to taste

Instructions:

1. In a saucepan, bring the chicken broth to a simmer over medium heat. Reduce heat to low to keep the broth warm.

2. In a large skillet, heat the olive oil over medium•high heat. Add the chicken and cook for 3•4 minutes until lightly browned. Remove chicken to a plate.

3. Add the mushrooms to the skillet and cook for 5 minutes until softened. Remove mushrooms to the plate with the chicken.

4. Reduce heat to medium and add the onion to the skillet. Cook for 3•4 minutes until translucent. Add the garlic and cook for 1 minute more.

5. Add the Arborio rice to the skillet and stir to coat with the oil. Cook for 2 minutes, stirring constantly.

6. Pour in the white wine and cook, stirring, until the wine is absorbed, about 2 minutes.

7. Ladle in 1/2 cup of the warm chicken broth and cook, stirring constantly, until the liquid is absorbed. Continue this process, adding 1/2 cup of broth at a time, until the rice is tender and creamy, about 20•25 minutes total.

8. Stir the cooked chicken and mushrooms back into the risotto. Remove from heat and stir in the Parmesan, butter, and parsley. Season with salt and pepper to taste. Serve the chicken and mushroom risotto immediately.

81. Beef and black bean chili

Ingredient:

• 1 lb ground beef
• 1 onion, diced
• 3 cloves garlic, minced
• 2 tbsp chili powder
• 1 tbsp ground cumin
• 1 tsp dried oregano
• 1 tsp smoked paprika
• 1/2 tsp cayenne pepper (optional, for heat)
• 1 (15 oz) can black beans, drained and rinsed
• 1 (15 oz) can diced tomatoes
• 1 (6 oz) can tomato paste
• 1 cup beef broth
• Salt and pepper to taste
• Toppings: shredded cheese, sour cream, chopped cilantro, etc.

Instructions:

1. In a large pot or Dutch oven, cook the ground beef over medium•high heat, breaking it up with a wooden spoon, until browned and cooked through, about 5•7 minutes. Drain excess fat.

2. Add the diced onion and cook for 3•4 minutes until softened. Add the garlic and cook for 1 minute more.

3. Stir in the chili powder, cumin, oregano, smoked paprika, and cayenne (if using). Cook for 1 minute to toast the spices.

4. Pour in the black beans, diced tomatoes, tomato paste, and beef broth. Stir to combine.

5. Bring the chili to a simmer, then reduce heat to medium•low. Let simmer for 20•30 minutes, stirring occasionally, until thickened.

6. Taste and season with salt and pepper as needed. Serve the beef and black bean chili hot, topped with desired toppings like shredded cheese, sour cream, and chopped cilantro.

This hearty chili is packed with bold Southwestern flavors from the spices and black beans. It's a perfect cold weather meal!

82. Chicken and corn chowder

Ingredient:

• 2 tbsp butter
• 1 onion, diced
• 2 celery stalks, diced
• 2 carrots, peeled and diced
• 3 cloves garlic, minced
• 1 lb boneless, skinless chicken breasts, cubed
• 4 cups chicken broth
• 2 medium potatoes, peeled and diced
• 2 cups frozen corn kernels
• 1 cup half•and•half or heavy cream
• 1 tsp dried thyme
• Salt and pepper to taste
• Chopped fresh parsley for garnish

Instructions:

1. In a large pot or Dutch oven, melt the butter over medium heat. Add the onion, celery, carrots and garlic. Cook for 5•7 minutes until vegetables are softened.

2. Add the cubed chicken to the pot and cook for 3•4 minutes, until chicken is lightly browned.

3. Pour in the chicken broth and add the diced potatoes. Bring to a boil, then reduce heat and simmer for 10•12 minutes, until potatoes are tender.

4. Stir in the frozen corn kernels and half•and•half. Season with the dried thyme, salt, and pepper.

5. Continue simmering for 5•10 more minutes, until chowder has thickened slightly.

6. Taste and adjust seasoning as needed.

7. Ladle the chicken and corn chowder into bowls and garnish with chopped fresh parsley.

Serve the chowder hot, with crusty bread on the side. The creamy broth, tender chicken, and sweet corn make this a comforting and satisfying meal.

83. Beef and barley soup

Ingredient:

- 2 lbs beef stew meat, cut into 1•inch cubes
- 2 tbsp olive oil
- 1 onion, diced
- 3 carrots, peeled and sliced
- 3 celery stalks, sliced
- 4 cloves garlic, minced
- 8 cups beef broth
- 1 cup pearl barley
- 1 (14.5 oz) can diced tomatoes
- 2 bay leaves
- 1 tsp dried thyme
- Salt and pepper to taste
- Chopped parsley for garnish

Instructions:

1. In a large pot or Dutch oven, heat the olive oil over medium•high heat. Add the beef cubes and brown on all sides, about 5 minutes total. Remove beef to a plate.

2. Add the onion, carrots, and celery to the pot. Cook for 5•7 minutes until vegetables are softened.

3. Stir in the garlic and cook for 1 minute.

4. Pour in the beef broth and add the browned beef back to the pot. Stir in the pearl barley, diced tomatoes, bay leaves, and thyme.

5. Bring the soup to a boil, then reduce heat to medium•low. Simmer for 45•60 minutes, until the beef is very tender and the barley is cooked through.

6. Remove the bay leaves. Taste the soup and season with salt and pepper as needed.

7. Ladle the beef and barley soup into bowls and garnish with chopped parsley.

Serve the soup hot, with crusty bread on the side. The tender beef, chewy barley, and hearty vegetables make this a satisfying and comforting meal.

84. Chicken and sweet potato curry

Ingredient:

- 1 lb boneless, skinless chicken thighs, cubed
- 2 tbsp olive oil
- 1 onion, diced
- 3 cloves garlic, minced
- 1 tbsp grated fresh ginger
- 2 tsp garam masala
- 1 tsp ground cumin
- 1 tsp ground coriander
- 1 tsp turmeric
- 1/4 tsp cayenne pepper (or to taste)
- 1 (14 oz) can diced tomatoes
- 1 (13.5 oz) can coconut milk
- 2 medium sweet potatoes, peeled and cubed
- 1 cup frozen peas
- Salt and pepper to taste
- Chopped cilantro for garnish

Instructions:

1. In a large skillet or Dutch oven, heat the olive oil over medium•high heat. Add the cubed chicken and cook for 5•7 minutes, until browned on all sides. Remove chicken from the pan and set aside.

2. In the same pan, add the diced onion and cook for 3•4 minutes until softened. Add the minced garlic and grated ginger and cook for 1 minute until fragrant.

3. Stir in the garam masala, cumin, coriander, turmeric, and cayenne pepper. Cook for 1 minute to toast the spices.

4. Pour in the diced tomatoes and coconut milk. Bring the mixture to a simmer.

5. Add the cubed sweet potatoes to the pan and return the cooked chicken to the curry. Reduce heat to medium•low, cover and simmer for 20•25 minutes, until the sweet potatoes are tender.

6. Stir in the frozen peas and cook for 5 more minutes.

7. Season the curry with salt and pepper to taste.

8. Serve the Chicken and Sweet Potato Curry over basmati rice, garnished with chopped cilantro.

The tender chicken and sweet potatoes are simmered in a rich, aromatic coconut milk•based curry sauce. It's a comforting and flavorful dish that pairs perfectly with the fluffy basmati rice. Enjoy!

85. Beef and vegetable curry

Ingredient:

- 1 lb beef stew meat, cut into 1•inch cubes
- 2 tbsp vegetable oil
- 1 onion, diced
- 3 cloves garlic, minced
- 1 tbsp grated fresh ginger
- 2 tbsp curry powder
- 1 tsp ground cumin
- 1 tsp ground coriander
- 1 tsp turmeric
- 1 tsp garam masala
- 1 (14 oz) can diced tomatoes
- 1 cup beef broth
- 1 cup coconut milk
- 2 medium potatoes, peeled and cubed
- 1 cup cauliflower florets
- 1 cup frozen peas
- Salt and pepper to taste
- Chopped cilantro for garnish
- Cooked basmati rice, for serving

Instructions:

1. In a large pot or Dutch oven, heat the vegetable oil over medium•high heat. Add the beef cubes and brown on all sides, about 5 minutes total. Remove beef to a plate.

2. Add the onion to the pot and cook for 5 minutes until softened. Add the garlic and ginger and cook for 1 minute.

3. Stir in the curry powder, cumin, coriander, turmeric, and garam masala. Cook for 1•2 minutes to toast the spices.

4. Pour in the diced tomatoes, beef broth, and coconut milk. Bring to a simmer.

5. Add the browned beef back to the pot along with the cubed potatoes, cauliflower florets, and frozen peas.

6. Reduce heat to medium•low, cover and simmer for 30•40 minutes, until beef and vegetables are very tender.

7. Taste and season with salt and pepper as needed. Serve the beef and vegetable curry over steamed basmati rice, garnished with chopped cilantro.

86. Chicken and vegetable kebabs

Ingredient:

• 1 lb boneless, skinless chicken breasts, cut into 1•inch cubes
• 1 red bell pepper, cut into 1•inch pieces
• 1 zucchini, cut into 1•inch slices
• 1 red onion, cut into 1•inch pieces
• 8 oz mushrooms, halved
• 2 tbsp olive oil
• 2 tbsp lemon juice
• 2 tsp dried oregano
• 1 tsp garlic powder
• Salt and pepper to taste
• Wooden or metal skewers

For Serving (optional):
• Lemon wedges
• Tzatziki sauce
• Pita bread

Instructions:

1. In a large bowl, combine the chicken, bell pepper, zucchini, onion, and mushrooms.

2. In a small bowl, whisk together the olive oil, lemon juice, oregano, garlic powder, salt, and pepper.

3. Pour the marinade over the chicken and vegetables and toss to coat everything evenly. Cover and refrigerate for 30 minutes to 1 hour.

4. Preheat grill or grill pan to medium•high heat.

5. Thread the marinated chicken and vegetables onto skewers, alternating the ingredients.

6. Grill the kebabs for 12•15 minutes, turning occasionally, until the chicken is cooked through and the vegetables are tender.

7. Serve the chicken and vegetable kebabs immediately, with lemon wedges, tzatziki sauce, and pita bread on the side if desired.

These colorful and flavorful kebabs are a great option for grilling. The chicken stays juicy and the vegetables get a nice char. Adjust the marinade ingredients to your taste preferences.

87. Beef and cheese enchiladas

Ingredient:

- 1 lb ground beef
- 1 onion, diced
- 2 cloves garlic, minced
- 1 tbsp chili powder
- 1 tsp ground cumin
- 1/2 tsp dried oregano
- Salt and pepper to taste
- 12 corn tortillas

- 2 cups shredded cheddar or Monterey Jack cheese
- 1 (15 oz) can enchilada sauce

For Serving (optional):
- Sour cream
- Diced tomatoes
- Chopped cilantro

Instructions:

1. Preheat oven to 350°F. Grease a 9x13 inch baking dish.

2. In a large skillet over medium·high heat, cook the ground beef, onion, and garlic until the beef is browned and crumbled, about 5·7 minutes. Drain any excess fat.

3. Stir in the chili powder, cumin, oregano, salt, and pepper. Cook for 1·2 minutes to toast the spices.

4. Warm the corn tortillas according to package instructions, or briefly in the microwave, to make them pliable.

5. Spread about 2·3 tbsp of the beef mixture down the center of each tortilla. Top with a sprinkle of shredded cheese.

6. Roll up the tortillas tightly and place seam·side down in the prepared baking dish.

7. Pour the enchilada sauce evenly over the top of the enchiladas. Sprinkle the remaining shredded cheese on top.

8. Bake for 20·25 minutes, until the cheese is melted and bubbly.

9. Serve the beef and cheese enchiladas warm, with optional toppings like sour cream, diced tomatoes, and chopped cilantro.

These hearty enchiladas are packed with seasoned ground beef and melty cheese. They make a delicious and comforting Tex·Mex meal.

88. Chicken and avocado wraps

Ingredient:

• 2 cups cooked, shredded chicken
• 1 avocado, diced
• 1/4 cup diced red onion
• 1/4 cup chopped fresh cilantro
• 2 tbsp lime juice
• 1 tsp olive oil
• 1/4 tsp salt
• 1/4 tsp black pepper
• 4•6 large tortilla or wrap shells

For Serving (optional):
• Shredded lettuce or spinach
• Diced tomatoes
• Shredded cheese
• Sour cream

Instructions:

1. In a medium bowl, combine the shredded chicken, diced avocado, red onion, cilantro, lime juice, olive oil, salt, and pepper. Stir gently to mix well.

2. Lay the tortilla or wrap shells out on a flat surface. Spoon an equal amount of the chicken and avocado mixture onto the center of each wrap.

3. If desired, top the chicken mixture with shredded lettuce or spinach, diced tomatoes, shredded cheese, and/or a dollop of sour cream.

4. Fold the bottom of the wrap up over the filling, then fold in the sides and continue rolling up tightly into a burrito shape.

5. Serve the chicken and avocado wraps immediately, or wrap in foil or parchment paper to enjoy later.

These wraps make a delicious and healthy lunch or light dinner. The creamy avocado, tender chicken, and fresh veggies are a winning combination. Adjust the fillings to your taste preferences.

Enjoy your homemade chicken and avocado wraps!

89. Beef and vegetable stir·fry

Ingredient:

- 1 lb beef sirloin or flank steak, thinly sliced
- 2 tbsp soy sauce, divided
- 1 tbsp cornstarch, divided
- 2 tbsp vegetable oil, divided
- 1 red bell pepper, sliced
- 1 cup broccoli florets
- 1 cup sliced mushrooms
- 1 cup snow peas or snap peas
- 3 cloves garlic, minced
- 1 tbsp grated fresh ginger
- 2 tbsp rice vinegar
- 1 tsp sesame oil
- Salt and pepper to taste
- Cooked rice, for serving

Instructions:

1. In a medium bowl, toss the sliced beef with 1 tbsp soy sauce and 1 tsp cornstarch until evenly coated. Set aside.

2. In a large skillet or wok, heat 1 tbsp vegetable oil over high heat. Add the bell pepper, broccoli, mushrooms, and snow peas. Stir·fry for 3·4 minutes until vegetables are crisp·tender. Remove vegetables to a plate.

3. Add the remaining 1 tbsp vegetable oil to the pan. Add the beef in a single layer and let sear for 1 minute without stirring. Flip the beef and sear the other side, about 1 minute more. Remove beef to the plate with the vegetables.

4. Reduce heat to medium and add the garlic and ginger to the pan. Cook for 30 seconds, stirring constantly, until fragrant.

5. In a small bowl, whisk together the remaining 1 tbsp soy sauce, 2 tsp cornstarch, rice vinegar, and sesame oil.

6. Pour the sauce mixture into the pan and let it simmer for 1·2 minutes until thickened slightly.

7. Return the beef and vegetables to the pan and toss everything together until heated through and coated in the sauce, about 2 minutes. Season with salt and pepper to taste. Serve the beef and vegetable stir·fry immediately over steamed rice.

90. Chicken and black bean burritos

Ingredient:

• 1 lb boneless, skinless chicken breasts, cooked and shredded
• 1 (15 oz) can black beans, drained and rinsed
• 1 cup cooked rice
• 1 cup shredded cheddar or Monterey Jack cheese
• 1/2 cup salsa
• 1 tsp ground cumin
• 1/2 tsp chili powder
• Salt and pepper to taste
• 8 large flour tortillas
• Optional toppings: sour cream, diced avocado, chopped cilantro

Instructions:

1. In a large bowl, combine the shredded chicken, black beans, cooked rice, shredded cheese, salsa, cumin, chili powder, salt, and pepper. Stir until well mixed.

2. Lay the flour tortillas out on a flat surface. Scoop about 1/2 cup of the chicken and bean mixture onto the center of each tortilla.

3. Fold the bottom of the tortilla up over the filling, then fold in the sides and continue rolling up tightly into a burrito shape.

4. Place the burritos seam•side down on a baking sheet or in a baking dish.

5. If baking immediately, preheat oven to 350°F. Bake the burritos for 15•20 minutes until heated through.

6. Alternatively, you can wrap the unbaked burritos individually in foil or parchment paper and freeze for later. To reheat, bake at 350°F for 25•30 minutes.

7. Serve the chicken and black bean burritos warm, with desired toppings like sour cream, diced avocado, and chopped cilantro.

These hearty burritos are packed with flavorful chicken, black beans, rice, and melty cheese. They make a satisfying and portable meal.

91. Beef and broccoli stir·fry

Ingredient:

- 1 lb flank steak or sirloin, thinly sliced against the grain
- 2 tbsp soy sauce, divided
- 1 tbsp cornstarch, divided
- 2 tbsp vegetable oil, divided
- 3 cups broccoli florets
- 3 cloves garlic, minced
- 1 tbsp grated fresh ginger
- 1/4 cup beef broth
- 2 tbsp brown sugar
- 1 tbsp rice vinegar
- 1 tsp sesame oil
- Salt and pepper to taste
- Cooked rice, for serving

Instructions:

1. In a medium bowl, toss the sliced beef with 1 tbsp soy sauce and 1 tsp cornstarch until evenly coated. Set aside.

2. In a large skillet or wok, heat 1 tbsp vegetable oil over high heat. Add the broccoli florets and stir·fry for 2·3 minutes until crisp·tender. Remove broccoli to a plate.

3. Add the remaining 1 tbsp vegetable oil to the pan. Add the beef in a single layer and let sear for 1 minute without stirring. Flip the beef and sear the other side, about 1 minute more. Remove beef to the plate with the broccoli.

4. Reduce heat to medium and add the garlic and ginger to the pan. Cook for 30 seconds, stirring constantly, until fragrant.

5. In a small bowl, whisk together the remaining 1 tbsp soy sauce, 2 tsp cornstarch, beef broth, brown sugar, rice vinegar, and sesame oil.

6. Pour the sauce mixture into the pan and let it simmer for 1·2 minutes until thickened slightly.

7. Return the beef and broccoli to the pan and toss everything together until heated through and coated in the sauce, about 2 minutes.

8. Season with salt and pepper to taste. Serve the beef and broccoli stir·fry immediately over steamed rice.

92. Chicken and pineapple fried rice

Ingredient:

• 2 cups cooked, diced chicken
• 2 tbsp vegetable oil
• 2 eggs, beaten
• 1 onion, diced
• 1 red bell pepper, diced
• 1 cup fresh pineapple chunks
• 3 cups cooked and chilled white rice
• 2 tbsp soy sauce
• 1 tsp sesame oil
• 1/2 tsp ground ginger
• Salt and pepper to taste
• Chopped green onions for garnish

Instructions:

1. Heat the vegetable oil in a large skillet or wok over medium•high heat.

2. Pour in the beaten eggs and scramble them, breaking them up into small pieces as they cook. Remove the eggs from the pan and set aside.

3. Add the diced onion and bell pepper to the hot pan. Stir•fry for 3•4 minutes until the vegetables are tender.

4. Add the diced chicken, pineapple chunks, and cooked rice to the pan. Stir to combine.

5. In a small bowl, whisk together the soy sauce, sesame oil, and ground ginger. Pour the sauce over the fried rice and toss everything together.

6. Allow the fried rice to cook for 2•3 minutes, stirring frequently, until heated through and the flavors have melded.

7. Stir the scrambled eggs back into the fried rice.

8. Season with salt and pepper to taste. Serve the chicken and pineapple fried rice hot, garnished with chopped green onions.

This sweet and savory fried rice dish is a delicious way to use up leftover chicken and rice. The pineapple adds a tropical twist that pairs perfectly with the soy•ginger sauce.

93. Beef and potato curry

Ingredient:

- 1 lb beef stew meat, cut into 1•inch cubes
- 2 tbsp vegetable oil
- 1 onion, diced
- 3 cloves garlic, minced
- 1 tbsp grated fresh ginger
- 2 tbsp curry powder
- 1 tsp ground cumin
- 1 tsp ground coriander
- 1 tsp turmeric
- 1 (14 oz) can diced tomatoes
- 1 cup beef broth
- 1 cup coconut milk
- 3 medium potatoes, peeled and cubed
- 1 cup frozen peas
- Salt and pepper to taste
- Chopped cilantro for garnish
- Cooked basmati rice, for serving

Instructions:

1. In a large pot or Dutch oven, heat the vegetable oil over medium•high heat. Add the beef cubes and brown on all sides, about 5 minutes total. Remove beef to a plate.

2. Add the diced onion to the pot and cook for 5 minutes until softened. Add the garlic and ginger and cook for 1 minute.

3. Stir in the curry powder, cumin, coriander, and turmeric. Cook for 1•2 minutes to toast the spices.

4. Pour in the diced tomatoes, beef broth, and coconut milk. Bring to a simmer.

5. Add the browned beef back to the pot along with the cubed potatoes.

6. Reduce heat to medium•low, cover and simmer for 30•40 minutes, until beef and potatoes are very tender.

7. Stir in the frozen peas and cook for 5 more minutes.

8. Taste and season with salt and pepper as needed.

9. Serve the beef and potato curry over steamed basmati rice, garnished with chopped cilantro.

This hearty curry is full of tender beef, creamy potatoes, and aromatic spices. It's a comforting and flavorful meal.

94. Chicken and vegetable curry

Ingredient:

- 1 tsp turmeric
- 1 (14 oz) can diced tomatoes
- 1 cup chicken broth
- 1 cup coconut milk
- 2 medium potatoes, peeled and cubed
- 1 cup cauliflower florets
- 1 cup frozen peas
- Salt and pepper to taste
- Chopped cilantro for garnish
- Cooked basmati rice, for serving

- 1 lb boneless, skinless chicken breasts, cut into 1•inch pieces
- 2 tbsp vegetable oil
- 1 onion, diced
- 3 cloves garlic, minced
- 1 tbsp grated fresh ginger
- 2 tbsp curry powder
- 1 tsp ground cumin
- 1 tsp ground coriander

Instructions:

1. In a large pot or Dutch oven, heat the vegetable oil over medium•high heat. Add the chicken pieces and cook for 3•4 minutes until lightly browned. Remove chicken to a plate.

2. Add the diced onion to the pot and cook for 5 minutes until softened. Add the garlic and ginger and cook for 1 minute.

3. Stir in the curry powder, cumin, coriander, and turmeric. Cook for 1•2 minutes to toast the spices.

4. Pour in the diced tomatoes, chicken broth, and coconut milk. Bring to a simmer.

5. Add the browned chicken back to the pot along with the cubed potatoes, cauliflower florets, and frozen peas.

6. Reduce heat to medium•low, cover and simmer for 20•25 minutes, until chicken and vegetables are tender.

7. Taste and season with salt and pepper as needed.

8. Serve the chicken and vegetable curry over steamed basmati rice, garnished with chopped cilantro.

This flavorful curry is packed with tender chicken, fresh vegetables, and aromatic spices. It's a comforting and satisfying meal.

95. Beef and cheese quesadillas

Ingredient:

- 1 lb ground beef
- 1 onion, diced
- 2 cloves garlic, minced
- 1 tbsp chili powder
- 1 tsp ground cumin
- 1/2 tsp dried oregano
- Salt and pepper to taste
- 8 medium flour tortillas
- 2 cups shredded cheddar or Monterey Jack cheese
- Sour cream, salsa, guacamole for serving (optional)

Instructions:

1. In a large skillet over medium•high heat, cook the ground beef, onion, and garlic until the beef is browned and crumbled, about 5•7 minutes. Drain any excess fat.

2. Stir in the chili powder, cumin, oregano, salt, and pepper. Cook for 1•2 minutes to toast the spices.

3. Lay 4 of the tortillas out on a flat surface. Divide the seasoned ground beef evenly among the tortillas, spreading it out to cover the surface.

4. Sprinkle the shredded cheese evenly over the beef on each tortilla.

5. Top each quesadilla with the remaining 4 tortillas, pressing down gently.

6. Heat a large skillet or griddle over medium heat. Working in batches if needed, cook the quesadillas for 2•3 minutes per side, until the tortillas are lightly browned and the cheese is melted.

7. Remove the quesadillas from the heat and cut each one into wedges.

8. Serve the beef and cheese quesadillas warm, with sour cream, salsa, and/or guacamole on the side for dipping, if desired.

These hearty quesadillas are packed with seasoned ground beef and melty cheese. They make a quick and satisfying meal or appetizer.

96. Chicken and vegetable stir·fry

Ingredient:

- 1 cup broccoli florets
- 1 cup sliced mushrooms
- 1 cup snow peas or snap peas
- 3 cloves garlic, minced
- 1 tbsp grated fresh ginger
- 2 tbsp rice vinegar
- 1 tsp sesame oil
- Salt and pepper to taste
- Cooked rice, for serving

- 1 lb boneless, skinless chicken breasts, cut into 1·inch pieces
- 2 tbsp soy sauce, divided
- 1 tbsp cornstarch, divided
- 2 tbsp vegetable oil, divided
- 1 red bell pepper, sliced

Instructions:

1. In a medium bowl, toss the chicken pieces with 1 tbsp soy sauce and 1 tsp cornstarch until evenly coated. Set aside.

2. In a large skillet or wok, heat 1 tbsp vegetable oil over high heat. Add the bell pepper, broccoli, mushrooms, and snow peas. Stir·fry for 3·4 minutes until vegetables are crisp·tender. Remove vegetables to a plate.

3. Add the remaining 1 tbsp vegetable oil to the pan. Add the chicken in a single layer and let sear for 1 minute without stirring. Flip the chicken and sear the other side, about 1 minute more. Remove chicken to the plate with the vegetables.

4. Reduce heat to medium and add the garlic and ginger to the pan. Cook for 30 seconds, stirring constantly, until fragrant.

5. In a small bowl, whisk together the remaining 1 tbsp soy sauce, 2 tsp cornstarch, rice vinegar, and sesame oil.

6. Pour the sauce mixture into the pan and let it simmer for 1·2 minutes until thickened slightly.

7. Return the chicken and vegetables to the pan and toss everything together until heated through and coated in the sauce, about 2 minutes.

8. Season with salt and pepper to taste. Serve the chicken and vegetable stir·fry immediately over steamed rice.

97. Beef and bean burritos

Ingredient:

- 1 lb ground beef
- 1 onion, diced
- 2 cloves garlic, minced
- 1 tbsp chili powder
- 1 tsp ground cumin
- 1 (15 oz) can black beans, drained and rinsed
- 1 cup cooked rice
- 1 cup shredded cheddar or Monterey Jack cheese
- 8 large flour tortillas
- Salsa, sour cream, guacamole for serving (optional)

Instructions:

1. In a large skillet over medium·high heat, cook the ground beef, onion, and garlic until the beef is browned and crumbled, about 5·7 minutes. Drain any excess fat.

2. Stir in the chili powder and cumin. Cook for 1·2 minutes to toast the spices.

3. Add the black beans and cooked rice to the skillet. Stir to combine and heat through.

4. Remove the skillet from heat and stir in the shredded cheese.

5. Lay the flour tortillas out on a flat surface. Scoop about 1/2 cup of the beef and bean mixture onto the center of each tortilla.

6. Fold the bottom of the tortilla up over the filling, then fold in the sides and continue rolling up tightly into a burrito shape.

7. Place the burritos seam·side down on a baking sheet or in a baking dish. If baking immediately, preheat oven to 350°F. Bake the burritos for 15·20 minutes until heated through.

8. Alternatively, you can wrap the unbaked burritos individually in foil or parchment paper and freeze for later. To reheat, bake at 350°F for 25·30 minutes.

9. Serve the beef and bean burritos warm, with salsa, sour cream, and guacamole on the side if desired.

These hearty burritos are packed with seasoned ground beef, black beans, rice, and melty cheese. They make a satisfying and portable meal.

98. Chicken and rice casserole

Ingredient:

• 1 lb boneless, skinless chicken breasts, cut into 1•inch pieces
• 1 cup uncooked long•grain white rice
• 1 (10.5 oz) can cream of mushroom soup
• 1 (10.5 oz) can cream of chicken soup
• 1 cup chicken broth
• 1/2 cup milk
• 1 tsp garlic powder
• 1 tsp onion powder
• 1/2 tsp dried thyme
• Salt and pepper to taste
• 1 cup frozen peas
• 1 cup shredded cheddar cheese

Instructions:

1. Preheat oven to 375°F. Grease a 9x13 inch baking dish.

2. In a large bowl, combine the chicken, uncooked rice, cream of mushroom soup, cream of chicken soup, chicken broth, milk, garlic powder, onion powder, thyme, salt and pepper. Mix well.

3. Spread the chicken and rice mixture evenly into the prepared baking dish. Cover tightly with foil.

4. Bake for 45 minutes. Remove foil, stir in the frozen peas, and sprinkle the shredded cheddar cheese on top.

5. Return to the oven and bake for 15 more minutes, until the rice is tender and the cheese is melted and bubbly.

6. Let stand for 5 minutes before serving.

Serve the chicken and rice casserole warm. Enjoy!

This is a simple, comforting one•dish meal that's perfect for busy weeknights. The creamy sauce, tender chicken, and cheesy topping make it a family favorite.

99. Beef and mushroom stroganoff

Ingredient:

- 1 lb beef sirloin or tenderloin, cut into 1•inch cubes
- 2 tbsp olive oil
- 1 onion, diced
- 8 oz mushrooms, sliced
- 2 cloves garlic, minced
- 1 tbsp tomato paste
- 1 cup beef broth
- 1/2 cup dry white wine or sherry
- 1 tsp Dijon mustard
- 1 tsp Worcestershire sauce
- 1 bay leaf
- 1 tsp paprika
- Salt and pepper to taste
- 1 cup sour cream
- 2 tbsp chopped fresh parsley
- Cooked egg noodles, for serving

Instructions:

1. In a large skillet, heat the olive oil over medium•high heat. Add the beef cubes and brown on all sides, about 5 minutes total. Remove beef to a plate.

2. Add the onions to the skillet and cook for 5 minutes until softened. Add the mushrooms and garlic and cook for 2•3 minutes more.

3. Stir in the tomato paste and cook for 1 minute.

4. Pour in the beef broth and white wine. Add the Dijon, Worcestershire, bay leaf, paprika, salt and pepper. Bring to a simmer.

5. Return the seared beef and any juices to the skillet. Reduce heat to low, cover and simmer for 45•60 minutes, until beef is very tender.

6. Remove the bay leaf. Stir in the sour cream and heat through, but do not boil.

7. Taste and adjust seasoning as needed. Stir in the chopped parsley.

8. Serve the beef stroganoff immediately over cooked egg noodles.

100. Chicken and broccoli Alfredo

Ingredient:

• 8 oz fettuccine pasta
• 1 lb boneless, skinless chicken breasts, cut into 1•inch pieces
• 2 tbsp olive oil
• 1 head broccoli, cut into florets
• 3 cloves garlic, minced
• 1 cup heavy cream
• 1 cup grated Parmesan cheese
• 2 tbsp butter
• 1/4 tsp nutmeg
• Salt and pepper to taste
• Chopped parsley for garnish

Instructions:

1. Bring a large pot of salted water to a boil. Cook the fettuccine according to package instructions until al dente. Drain and set aside.

2. In a large skillet, heat the olive oil over medium•high heat. Add the chicken pieces and cook for 5•7 minutes, until browned on all sides and cooked through. Remove chicken to a plate.

3. In the same skillet, add the broccoli florets and a splash of water. Cover and steam the broccoli for 3•4 minutes until tender•crisp. Remove broccoli to the plate with the chicken.

4. Reduce heat to medium and add the minced garlic to the skillet. Cook for 1 minute, stirring constantly, until fragrant.

5. Pour in the heavy cream and whisk in the Parmesan cheese. Bring the sauce to a simmer and cook for 2•3 minutes, until thickened slightly.

6. Stir the cooked fettuccine, chicken, and broccoli into the Alfredo sauce. Add the butter and nutmeg. Toss everything together until well coated.

7. Season with salt and pepper to taste.

8. Serve the chicken and broccoli Alfredo immediately, garnished with chopped parsley.

This creamy, cheesy pasta dish is a delicious way to enjoy chicken and broccoli. The Alfredo sauce ties all the flavors together perfectly.

101. Beef and potato stew

Ingredient:

- 2 lbs beef stew meat, cut into 1•inch cubes
- 3 tablespoons olive oil
- 1 large onion, diced
- 3 cloves garlic, minced
- 2 tablespoons tomato paste
- 1 cup red wine or beef broth
- 4 cups beef broth
- 2 bay leaves
- 1 teaspoon dried thyme
- Salt and pepper to taste
- 3 medium potatoes, peeled and cut into 1•inch cubes
- 2 carrots, peeled and sliced
- 1 cup frozen peas

Instructions:

1. In a large pot or Dutch oven, heat the olive oil over medium•high heat. Add the beef cubes and brown on all sides, about 5 minutes total. Remove beef to a plate.

2. Add the onion to the pot and cook for 5 minutes until softened. Add the garlic and tomato paste and cook for 1 minute.

3. Pour in the red wine (or beef broth) and use a wooden spoon to scrape up any browned bits from the bottom of the pot.

4. Add the beef back to the pot along with the beef broth, bay leaves, thyme, salt and pepper. Bring to a boil.

5. Reduce heat to low, cover and simmer for 1 hour.

6. Add the potatoes and carrots. Cover and simmer for 30•40 minutes more, until beef and vegetables are very tender.

7. Stir in the frozen peas and cook for 5 more minutes.

8. Taste and adjust seasoning as needed.

9. Serve the beef and potato stew hot

102. Chicken and spinach lasagna

Ingredient:

• 9 lasagna noodles
• 2 cups cooked, shredded chicken
• 1 (10 oz) package frozen chopped spinach, thawed and drained
• 1 (15 oz) container ricotta cheese
• 2 cups shredded mozzarella cheese, divided
• 1/2 cup grated Parmesan cheese
• 2 eggs
• 1 tsp dried basil
• 1/2 tsp garlic powder
• 1/4 tsp nutmeg
• Salt and pepper to taste
• 1 (24 oz) jar marinara sauce

Instructions:

1. Preheat oven to 375°F. Grease a 9x13 inch baking dish.

2. Bring a large pot of salted water to a boil. Cook the lasagna noodles according to package instructions until al dente. Drain and set aside.

3. In a medium bowl, mix together the shredded chicken, drained spinach, ricotta, 1 cup of the mozzarella, Parmesan, eggs, basil, garlic powder, nutmeg, salt and pepper.

4. Spread 1 cup of the marinara sauce in the bottom of the prepared baking dish.

5. Arrange 3 lasagna noodles in a single layer over the sauce. Spread half of the chicken•spinach mixture over the noodles.

6. Top with another layer of 3 noodles, the remaining chicken•spinach mixture, and 1 cup of the marinara sauce.

7. Top with the final 3 noodles and the remaining marinara sauce.

8. Sprinkle the remaining 1 cup of mozzarella cheese over the top.

9. Cover with foil and bake for 40 minutes. Remove foil and bake for 10•15 minutes more, until cheese is melted and bubbly. Let the lasagna stand for 10 minutes before serving.

Serve the chicken and spinach lasagna warm. This creamy, cheesy lasagna is a delicious way to use up leftover chicken. The spinach adds a nice nutritional boost.

103. Beef and vegetable stir·fry

Ingredient:

- 1 cup sliced mushrooms
- 1 cup snow peas or snap peas
- 3 cloves garlic, minced
- 1 tbsp grated fresh ginger
- 2 tbsp rice vinegar
- 1 tsp sesame oil
- Salt and pepper to taste
- Cooked rice, for serving

- 1 lb beef sirloin or flank steak, thinly sliced
- 2 tbsp soy sauce, divided
- 1 tbsp cornstarch, divided
- 2 tbsp vegetable oil, divided
- 1 red bell pepper, sliced
- 1 cup broccoli florets

Instructions:

1. In a medium bowl, toss the sliced beef with 1 tbsp soy sauce and 1 tsp cornstarch until evenly coated. Set aside.

2. In a large skillet or wok, heat 1 tbsp vegetable oil over high heat. Add the bell pepper, broccoli, mushrooms, and snow peas. Stir·fry for 3·4 minutes until vegetables are crisp·tender. Remove vegetables to a plate.

3. Add the remaining 1 tbsp vegetable oil to the pan. Add the beef in a single layer and let sear for 1 minute without stirring. Flip the beef and sear the other side, about 1 minute more. Remove beef to the plate with the vegetables.

4. Reduce heat to medium and add the garlic and ginger to the pan. Cook for 30 seconds, stirring constantly, until fragrant.

5. In a small bowl, whisk together the remaining 1 tbsp soy sauce, 2 tsp cornstarch, rice vinegar, and sesame oil.

6. Pour the sauce mixture into the pan and let it simmer for 1·2 minutes until thickened slightly.

7. Return the beef and vegetables to the pan and toss everything together until heated through and coated in the sauce, about 2 minutes.

8. Season with salt and pepper to taste. Serve the beef and vegetable stir·fry immediately over steamed rice.

104. Chicken and mushroom risotto

Ingredient:

• 4 cups chicken broth
• 2 tbsp olive oil
• 1 lb boneless, skinless chicken breasts, cut into 1•inch pieces
• 8 oz cremini or button mushrooms, sliced
• 1 onion, diced
• 2 cloves garlic, minced
• 1 1/2 cups Arborio rice
• 1/2 cup dry white wine
• 1/2 cup grated Parmesan cheese
• 2 tbsp butter
• 2 tbsp chopped fresh parsley
• Salt and pepper to taste

Instructions:

1. In a saucepan, bring the chicken broth to a simmer over medium heat. Reduce heat to low to keep the broth warm.

2. In a large skillet, heat the olive oil over medium•high heat. Add the chicken and cook for 3•4 minutes until lightly browned. Remove chicken to a plate.

3. Add the mushrooms to the skillet and cook for 5 minutes until softened. Remove mushrooms to the plate with the chicken.

4. Reduce heat to medium and add the onion to the skillet. Cook for 3•4 minutes until translucent. Add the garlic and cook for 1 minute more.

5. Add the Arborio rice to the skillet and stir to coat with the oil. Cook for 2 minutes, stirring constantly.

6. Pour in the white wine and cook, stirring, until the wine is absorbed, about 2 minutes.

7. Ladle in 1/2 cup of the warm chicken broth and cook, stirring constantly, until the liquid is absorbed. Continue this process, adding 1/2 cup of broth at a time, until the rice is tender and creamy, about 20•25 minutes total.

8. Stir the cooked chicken and mushrooms back into the risotto. Remove from heat and stir in the Parmesan, butter, and parsley. Season with salt and pepper to taste. Serve the chicken and mushroom risotto immediately

105. Beef and black bean chili

Ingredient:

- 1 lb ground beef
- 1 onion, diced
- 3 cloves garlic, minced
- 2 tbsp chili powder
- 1 tbsp ground cumin
- 1 tsp dried oregano
- 1 tsp smoked paprika
- 1/2 tsp cayenne pepper (optional, for heat)
- 1 (15 oz) can black beans, drained and rinsed
- 1 (15 oz) can diced tomatoes
- 1 (6 oz) can tomato paste
- 1 cup beef broth
- Salt and pepper to taste
- Toppings: shredded cheese, sour cream, chopped cilantro, etc.

Instructions:

1. In a large pot or Dutch oven, cook the ground beef over medium•high heat, breaking it up with a wooden spoon, until browned and cooked through, about 5•7 minutes. Drain excess fat.

2. Add the diced onion and cook for 3•4 minutes until softened. Add the garlic and cook for 1 minute more.

3. Stir in the chili powder, cumin, oregano, smoked paprika, and cayenne (if using). Cook for 1 minute to toast the spices.

4. Pour in the black beans, diced tomatoes, tomato paste, and beef broth. Stir to combine.

5. Bring the chili to a simmer, then reduce heat to medium•low. Let simmer for 20•30 minutes, stirring occasionally, until thickened.

6. Taste and season with salt and pepper as needed. Serve the beef and black bean chili hot, topped with desired toppings like shredded cheese, sour cream, and chopped cilantro.

This hearty chili is packed with bold Southwestern flavors from the spices and black beans. It's a perfect cold weather meal!

106. Chicken and corn chowder

Ingredient:

• 2 tablespoons olive oil
• 1 onion, diced
• 2 carrots, peeled and diced
• 2 celery stalks, diced
• 3 cloves garlic, minced
• 4 cups chicken broth
• 2 medium potatoes, peeled and diced
• 2 cups cooked chicken, shredded or cubed
• 2 cups frozen corn kernels
• 1 cup half•and•half or heavy cream
• 1 teaspoon dried thyme
• Salt and pepper to taste
• Chopped parsley for garnish (optional)

Instructions:

1. In a large pot or Dutch oven, heat the olive oil over medium heat. Add the onion, carrots, celery and garlic. Cook for 5•7 minutes until the vegetables are softened.

2. Pour in the chicken broth and add the diced potatoes. Bring to a boil, then reduce heat and simmer for 10•15 minutes until the potatoes are tender.

3. Stir in the cooked chicken, corn, half•and•half or cream, and thyme. Season with salt and pepper to taste.

4. Simmer the chowder for 5•10 more minutes to allow the flavors to meld.

5. Ladle the chowder into bowls and garnish with chopped parsley if desired.

Enjoy your hearty and comforting chicken and corn chowder!

107. Beef and barley soup

Ingredient:

- 2 lbs beef stew meat, cut into 1•inch cubes
- 2 tablespoons olive oil
- 1 onion, diced
- 3 carrots, peeled and diced
- 3 celery stalks, diced
- 4 cloves garlic, minced
- 8 cups beef broth
- 1 cup pearl barley
- 1 (14.5 oz) can diced tomatoes
- 2 bay leaves
- 1 teaspoon dried thyme
- Salt and pepper to taste
- Chopped parsley for garnish (optional)

Instructions:

1. In a large pot or Dutch oven, heat the olive oil over medium•high heat. Add the beef cubes and brown on all sides, about 5 minutes total. Remove beef to a plate.

2. Add the onion, carrots, celery and garlic to the pot. Cook for 5•7 minutes until the vegetables are softened.

3. Pour in the beef broth and add the browned beef, pearl barley, diced tomatoes, bay leaves and thyme. Season with salt and pepper.

4. Bring the soup to a boil, then reduce heat and let it simmer for 45•60 minutes, until the beef is very tender and the barley is cooked through.

5. Remove the bay leaves. Taste and adjust seasoning as needed.

6. Ladle the beef and barley soup into bowls and garnish with chopped parsley if desired.

This hearty and comforting soup is perfect for a chilly day. The beef and barley make it nice and filling. Enjoy!

108. Chicken and sweet potato curry

Ingredient:

• 1 lb boneless, skinless chicken thighs, cut into 1•inch pieces
• 2 tablespoons olive oil
• 1 onion, diced
• 3 cloves garlic, minced
• 1 tablespoon grated fresh ginger
• 2 teaspoons curry powder
• 1 teaspoon ground cumin
• 1 teaspoon ground coriander
• 1/4 teaspoon cayenne pepper (or more to taste)
• 1 (14 oz) can coconut milk
• 2 cups chicken broth
• 2 medium sweet potatoes, peeled and cubed
• 1 cup frozen peas
• Salt and pepper to taste
• Chopped cilantro for garnish

Instructions:

1. In a large pot or Dutch oven, heat the olive oil over medium•high heat. Add the chicken and cook for 3•4 minutes until lightly browned. Remove chicken to a plate.

2. Add the onion to the pot and cook for 5 minutes until softened. Add the garlic, ginger, curry powder, cumin, coriander and cayenne. Cook for 1 minute until fragrant.

3. Pour in the coconut milk and chicken broth. Bring to a simmer, then add the cubed sweet potatoes. Reduce heat to medium•low and let simmer for 15•20 minutes until the sweet potatoes are tender.

4. Stir the cooked chicken and frozen peas into the curry. Simmer for 5 more minutes until the chicken is cooked through.

5. Season the curry with salt and pepper to taste.

6. Serve the chicken and sweet potato curry over basmati rice. Garnish with chopped cilantro.

This curry is full of warm spices, tender chicken, and sweet potatoes. It's a comforting and flavorful dish that's perfect for a chilly evening. Enjoy!

109. Beef and vegetable curry

Ingredient:

- 1 lb beef stew meat, cut into 1·inch cubes
- 2 tablespoons olive oil
- 1 onion, diced
- 3 cloves garlic, minced
- 1 tablespoon grated fresh ginger
- 2 tablespoons curry powder
- 1 teaspoon ground cumin
- 1 teaspoon ground coriander
- 1/4 teaspoon cayenne pepper (or more to taste)
- 1 (14 oz) can coconut milk
- 1 cup beef broth
- 2 medium potatoes, peeled and cubed
- 2 carrots, peeled and sliced
- 1 cup frozen peas
- Salt and pepper to taste
- Chopped cilantro for garnish

Instructions:

1. In a large pot or Dutch oven, heat the olive oil over medium·high heat. Add the beef cubes and brown on all sides, about 5 minutes total. Remove beef to a plate.

2. Add the onion to the pot and cook for 5 minutes until softened. Add the garlic, ginger, curry powder, cumin, coriander and cayenne. Cook for 1 minute until fragrant.

3. Pour in the coconut milk and beef broth. Bring to a simmer, then add the cubed potatoes and sliced carrots. Reduce heat to medium·low and let simmer for 15·20 minutes until the vegetables are tender.

4. Stir the browned beef and frozen peas into the curry. Simmer for 10 more minutes until the beef is cooked through.

5. Season the curry with salt and pepper to taste.

6. Serve the beef and vegetable curry over basmati rice. Garnish with chopped cilantro.

This hearty curry is packed with tender beef, potatoes, carrots, and peas in a rich coconut milk·based sauce. The blend of warm spices makes it extra flavorful. Enjoy!

110. Chicken and vegetable kebabs

Ingredient:

• 1 lb boneless, skinless chicken breasts, cut into 1•inch cubes
• 1 red bell pepper, cut into 1•inch pieces
• 1 yellow bell pepper, cut into 1•inch pieces
• 1 red onion, cut into 1•inch pieces
• 8 oz mushrooms, halved
• 1 zucchini, cut into 1•inch pieces
• 2 tablespoons olive oil
• 2 tablespoons lemon juice
• 2 teaspoons dried oregano
• 1 teaspoon garlic powder
• Salt and pepper to taste
• Wooden or metal skewers

Marinade:
• 1/4 cup olive oil
• 2 tablespoons lemon juice
• 2 cloves garlic, minced
• 1 teaspoon dried oregano
• 1/2 teaspoon salt
• 1/4 teaspoon black pepper

Instructions:

1. In a large bowl, whisk together the marinade ingredients. Add the chicken cubes and toss to coat. Cover and refrigerate for 30 minutes to 1 hour.

2. In a separate bowl, toss the chopped vegetables with the 2 tablespoons olive oil, 2 tablespoons lemon juice, 2 teaspoons oregano, garlic powder, salt and pepper.

3. Preheat grill to medium•high heat.

4. Thread the marinated chicken and seasoned vegetables onto skewers, alternating between the ingredients.

5. Grill the kebabs for 12•15 minutes, turning occasionally, until the chicken is cooked through and the vegetables are tender.

6. Serve the chicken and vegetable kebabs immediately, with any extra marinade drizzled over the top